LASIK

A Guide to Laser Vision Correction

ERNEST W. KORNMEHL, M.D.

ROBERT K. MALONEY, M.D.

JONATHAN M. DAVIDORF, M.D.

ADDICUS BOOKS
OMAHA, NEBRASKA

An Addicus Nonfiction Book

ISBN 1-886039-54-2
Cover design by Jack Kusler and Peri Poloni
Color illustrations by Mary Bryson
Black-and-white illustrations by Jack Kusler

This book is not intended to serve as a substitute for a physician, nor do the authors intend to give medical advice contrary to that of an attending physician.

Library of Congress Cataloging-in-Publication Data

Kornmehl, Ernest W., 1959-
   Lasik : a guide to laser vision correction / Ernest W. Kornmehl,
Robert K. Maloney, Jonathan M. Davidorf.
      p. cm.
Includes bibliographical references and index.
   ISBN 1-886039-54-2
   1. LASIK (Eye surgery)—Popular works. I. Davidorf, Jonathan M.,
1965- II. Maloney, Robert K., 1958- III. Title.
   RE336 .K67 2001
   617.7'1—dc21

                                                                2001003385

Addicus Books, Inc.
P.O. Box 45327
Omaha, Nebraska 68145
Web site: http://www.AddicusBooks.com
Printed in the United States of America
10 9 8 7 6 5 4 3 2 1

Contents

Acknowledgments

I would like to thank my wife Ellen Kornmehl, M.D., for her support of my efforts with this book; she is my role model for a caring, compassionate physician. I would also like to acknowledge my parents, Nathan and Frances Kornmehl, for teaching me that being a physician is a privilege and position of trust that can never be violated. I thank Melinda Jordan for her editorial help and for her assistance in developing a world-class laser center; I also wish to express my gratitude to the entire staff of the Kornmehl Laser Eye Associates for the extraordinary care they provide our patients. Finally, I am grateful to the thousands of patients, and the doctors who referred them, for entrusting me with their most precious sense— the gift of sight.

Ernest W. Kornmehl, M.D.

I wish to thank my father, who taught me to be uncompromising in the pursuit of excellence, and my mother, who taught me that great relationships require compromise. I particularly thank my fabulous wife, Nicole, for her patience with the demands of my chosen career. At times, she must wish that I had listened more to my mother's advice.

Robert K. Maloney, M.D.

I would like to thank my father, Dr. Bernard Davidorf, for introducing me to ophthalmology and my mother, Eleanor Davidorf, for teaching me the importance of listening to my patients. I also wish to thank my uncle, Dr. Frederick Davidorf, for encouraging me in my research endeavors and for teaching me the importance of communicating new ideas through scientific publication. I thank Dr. Roberto Zaldivar, my mentor in the field of refractive surgery. Most importantly, my deep appreciation goes to my wife Jaime and our two children, Carolena and Benjamin, for their energizing spirits, support, and understanding.

Jonathan M. Davidorf, M.D.

Introduction

Just about everyone knows someone who has had laser vision correction. That's not surprising when you consider that more than 1.3 million LASIK procedures are performed annually in the United States. As the number of these procedures continues to grow exponentially, so, it seems, does the hype. Advertisements, articles, web sites, and patient testimonials abound. Exciting as this technology is, there's a lot of misinformation that can be confusing to those considering laser vision correction.

Why, for example, does one center offer laser vision correction for half the price of another center? And what is the consumer to make of ads claiming you can "Throw your eyeglasses away for good!" and "Get 20/20 vision—guaranteed"? A smart consumer considering laser vision correction needs to become well informed. It is essential that you arm yourself with unbiased, complete information before undergoing such a procedure.

That's why we embarked on this book: to provide you with an easy-to-understand, thorough, and accurate educational tool that will answer your questions about one of the most popular surgical procedures—LASIK vision correction. We are committed to helping people understand the real—not the hyped—benefits of LASIK, as well as its disadvantages and potential risks.

If you are contemplating laser vision correction, you will want to know whether you are a good candidate for LASIK. You will need to find out exactly what is involved, how the procedure works, and how much it costs. You will also want to know what kind of eyesight you can reasonably expect after the surgery, as well as all the possible risks and complications. And you may need guidance on choosing a qualified laser surgeon—someone you can really trust. It is our intent to provide this kind of information in our book.

In our medical practices, we talk to thousands of patients each year. When it comes to LASIK, similar questions come up again and again. We kept these questions in mind as we worked on this book. We are also familiar with and understand the kinds of anxieties and misconceptions most patients have when they enter our offices for the first time. It is our hope that we can relieve your fears by educating you about LASIK.

1

The Human Eye and How Vision Works

S ight is often considered the most precious of our senses. Our eyes enable us to take in the surrounding world. Without sight, the way we perceive the world would be forever changed. No wonder the eyes are often elevated in literature, art, religion, and philosophy to symbolize everything from the windows of the soul to Supreme Wisdom. Indeed, the eyes are a marvel of mechanics.

However, changes within the eyeball may occur, resulting in impaired vision. Objects that we once viewed with crystal clarity may become blurred or distorted. To better understand how our vision may change, let's first examine the anatomy of the eyeball.

How the Eye Works

You may have heard the comparison between a camera and the human eye. Just as a camera takes in light and transforms it into an image on film, your eye does virtually the same thing, only the "film" is your retina and your brain "develops" the image. We see objects when light, which is reflected by the objects, passes through the eyeball lens and strikes the retina at the back of the eye. Our brains then interpret the shapes, colors, and dimensions of the objects we see. A clearly focused object is the result of normal vision. However, just as an improper amount of light entering a camera lens will distort a photo, if light entering the eyeball does not strike the retina the result may be distorted vision.

Anatomy of the Eye

Sclera and Cornea

The outer layer surrounding the eyeball is made up of two parts: the *sclera* and the *cornea*. The sclera—the white, opaque part of the eye—makes up the back five-sixths of the eye's outer layer and provides protection for the eyeball. The cornea, about the size of a dime and as thick as a credit card, makes up the remaining one-sixth of the eye's outer layer. It is the transparent, dome-shaped bulge at the front of the eyeball. The cornea provides most of the eye's focusing power, so small changes in its curvature can make an enormous difference in how clearly you see objects.

The cornea has three main layers. The *epithelium* is the thin outer protective layer of cells; it is made up of the same kind of tissue that covers most of your body, and is continually regenerating, or renewing itself. The *stroma* is the strong, fibrous layer that makes up 90 percent of the cornea's thickness and provides the cornea with its structure and shape. The *endothelium* is the single cell layer that lines the inside of the cornea and helps regulate the cornea's fluid content.

Iris

The *iris*, which determines one's eye color, is located behind the cornea. It is composed of connective tissue and smooth

The Eyeball

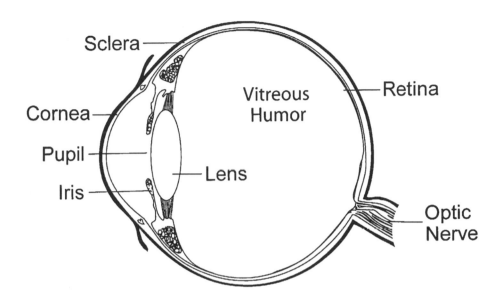

muscle fibers. The muscles of the iris control how much light passes through to the retina.

Pupil

The *pupil* appears as a black circle in the middle of the iris. The pupil can be likened to the aperture, or shutter, of a camera. When it is very bright, as on a sunny day, the iris muscles make the pupil *constrict,* or become small, so only a small amount of light will pass into the eye. In darkness the opposite happens, and the pupil *dilates,* or enlarges, to let in more light.

Lens

The *lens* is a circular structure located directly behind the pupil and held in place by slender, strong ligaments. Although most of the bending of light is accomplished by the cornea, the curved lens fine-tunes the angle of light passing through it, focusing the light onto the retina. When the ligaments tighten, the lens becomes flatter, or less convex, allowing you to see objects at a distance. When the ligaments relax, the elastic lens becomes rounder, or more convex (like a magnifying glass), so you can see objects that are close. This ability of the lens to refine the focus through flexing is called *accommodation*.

Normal Vision

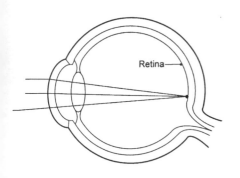

When one has normal vision, light rays enter through the lens and strike the retina, producing a focused image.

Vitreous Humor

The *vitreous humor* is the gel-like substance, about 99 percent water, that fills the space between the lens and the retina on the inner back wall of the eye. Light passes through the vitreous humor before striking the retina.

Retina

The *retina* is a complex layer of nerve tissue that lines the inside back wall of the eyeball. Similar to film in a camera, the retina "captures" the image through an electrochemical reaction to light. Electrical impulses are then transmitted through the *optic nerve* to the brain, which interprets or "develops" the image.

Common Vision Problems

Your eye doctor may refer to your vision problem as your *refractive error,* or focusing problem. How well you see is determined, for the most part, by how accurately your eyes are able to bend, or *refract,* light. In a normal eye, the focus comes to a point on the retina. But sometimes this does not occur. The result? Various forms of vision impairment. Below are some common refractive errors, or vision problems.

Myopia (Nearsightedness)

Myopia

Also known as *nearsightedness, myopia* is a condition in which you can see nearby objects well, but objects at a distance appear blurred. This happens when light bouncing off a faraway image enters the eye through the cornea and comes to a point of focus too soon, before it reaches the retina. Myopia may be due to a cornea that has too much curvature, which causes the light to "overbend" and focus in front of the retina. Myopia also occurs when the eyeball is too long—the retinal wall is too far back for the combined focusing power of the cornea and lens.

In myopia, or nearsightedness, light rays focus in front of the retina, causing distant objects to appear blurry.

Hyperopia (Farsightedness)

People with *hyperopia,* or *farsightedness,* see distant objects more clearly than nearby objects when they are young but may have difficulty with both as they get older. In hyperopia, the light

Hyperopia

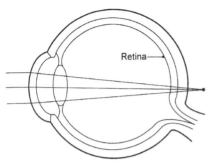

In hyperopia, or farsightedness, light rays focus behind the retina. Objects in the distance are seen more clearly than near objects.

rays coming into the cornea are not bent sharply enough, and are focused behind, rather than on, the retina. The result is a blurred image. This usually happens in people whose eyeballs are too short from front to back, or whose focusing muscles around the lens are too weak. Another cause of hyperopia, though rare, is a cornea that is too flat.

Because muscles are more elastic in youth, younger people who are mildly hyperopic can actually compensate for it by using the focusing muscles around the lens to fine-tune the focus by bending light more steeply. This action brings the point of focus forward toward the retina, allowing them to see more clearly. However, since the muscles weaken and the lens becomes less pliable as we age, these individuals eventually lose that ability and may no longer see well at a distance or close up. After age forty, they may be completely dependent on eyeglasses or contact lenses for both close and distant vision.

Astigmatism

Many individuals with myopia or hyperopia also have some degree of *astigmatism*. People with significant astigmatism experience blurred or distorted vision for all objects, whether near or far. Astigmatism means that your cornea, instead of being spherical like the side of a basketball, is slightly oval, shaped more like the side of a football. As a result, light rays entering the eye from different points on the cornea's surface are bent irregularly and are focused at several different points, rather than meeting at just one focal point. Almost everyone has a small degree of astigmatism.

Presbyopia

Farsightedness is often confused with *presbyopia* (literally, "old eyes"). Presbyopia is the age-dependent need for reading glasses or bifocals. After age forty, and usually by age forty-five in most people, the ability to focus on an object close up, such as a restaurant menu, becomes more difficult. This happens to most everyone. It is due to a loss of flexibility in the lens and a weakening in the muscles that enable the lens to flex and fine-tune the focus. Presbyopia typically continues to worsen until age sixty-five. When this occurs, people who already wear eyeglasses may need bifocals, and those who have never worn eyeglasses may require reading glasses.

Astigmatism

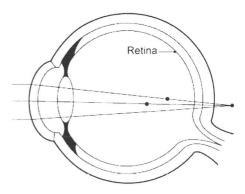

In astigmatism, light entering the eyeball focuses on multiple areas rather than on the retina. Objects both far and near appear blurry.

How Your Vision Is Measured

Most people who have had an eye exam that includes a test to measure *visual acuity* (the clarity or sharpness of one's vision) recognize the simple notation 20/20 as meaning "normal vision." What do those numbers mean? Let's say your vision is 20/40. That means you can see at twenty feet what a person with normal vision can see at forty feet. Your measure of visual acuity is determined by using the *Snellen chart,* that familiar eye chart with progressively smaller letters on each line. Although it is considered an accurate vision test, the results are sometimes affected by such variables as squinting, guessing at the letters, and room light.

So, numbers such as 20/20 or 20/40 describe your visual acuity but do not measure your refractive error—how accurately your eye bends, or refracts, light. When an eye doctor measures your refractive error, what you end up with is your eyeglass prescription. Finding an eye doctor whose measurements are impeccable is crucial, not just for your eyeglass prescription, but also, as you will learn later, for laser vision correction.

Understanding Your Eyeglass Prescription

Your eyeglass prescription is written in numbers. The type and degree of refractive error is quantified in units of measure called *diopters*. If you have ever wondered what those numbers mean, here is how to read and understand your prescription.

To arrive at your prescription, your doctor takes three measurements during the eye exam: sphere, cylinder, and axis. Your prescription for glasses may look something like this:

Right   -1.25   —   —

Left   -1.25   -.25   X   170

The first number represents the *sphere*. The sphere measure tells the eye doctor where your eye focuses light: on the retina (normal vision), in front of the retina (myopia), or behind the retina (hyperopia). In other words, the sphere measure reveals whether you are nearsighted or farsighted. A negative diopter indicates myopia, or nearsightedness. A positive diopter indicates hyperopia, or farsightedness. The higher the number, the stronger the prescription. In the example above, the person has mild myopia (-1.25 diopters) in both eyes.

The second number represents the *cylinder*. The cylinder measure indicates whether the patient has astigmatism. A number in the cylinder column means some degree of astigmatism is present. The larger the number, the more severe the astigmatism. The example above reveals that this person has no astigmatism in the right eye, and a small amount (-.25 diopter) in the left eye.

If astigmatism is present, your eye doctor takes an *axis* measurement. The axis measure indicates where irregularity lies on the eyeball. In the prescription above, the astigmatism in the left eye is positioned at the 170-degree axis.

Diopter Ranges for Refractive Errors

Type of Refractive Error	Mild	Moderate	Severe	Extreme
Myopia	less than –3.00	–3.00 to –6.00	–6.00 to –9.00	Greater than –9.00
Hyperopia	+1.00 to +1.25	+1.50 to +3.50	+3.75 to +5.00	Greater than +5.00
Astigmatism	less than 1.00	1.00 to 2.25	2.25 to 3.00	Greater than 3.00

Nonsurgical Vision Correction Options

Eyeglasses

Eyeglasses have been around for hundreds of years. As early as the thirteenth century, inventors in China and Europe inserted magnifiers into frames, making the first prototype for our modern-day eyeglasses. Like the early versions, today's eyeglasses work like magnifying glasses that enhance the eye's ability to focus sharply, whether near or far. The amount of curvature in the spectacle lens determines how light bends before it reaches your cornea. Vision is corrected, depending on the angle of refraction, to compensate for your focusing error.

Eyeglasses have a number of advantages. They are usually affordable, easy to maintain, and can be adapted for a number of different uses, such as reading, active sports, and driving. They also have disadvantages. Eyeglasses may restrict *peripheral vision* (the outer part of your field of vision), prove difficult in certain weather conditions such as rain or snow, and make images appear smaller or larger than they really are. They may cause a number of visual aberrations (including halos around lights) and have a limited usage life. Eyeglasses may interfere with certain occupations and recreational activities—swimming, for example. And some people just don't like the way they look in eyeglasses.

Contact Lenses

Contact lenses offer another option for correcting vision. Like eyeglasses, they make up the difference between the amount of refraction your eye can accomplish on its own and what is needed for sharp focus. Because they are extremely thin and custom shaped for your cornea, contact lenses float on the surface of your eye; they are held in place by natural suction and are constantly lubricated by the eye's own moisture.

Contact lenses have some advantages over eyeglasses. For example, contacts enable the wearer to have more natural vision (including better peripheral vision), cause little noticeable change in cosmetic appearance, and allow more freedom in recreational activities. On the other hand, contacts require maintenance—continuous, frequent cleaning. Users must buy cleaning and storage solutions. The lenses may tear easily. They may be inconvenient for traveling, and also are easily lost. Contacts may be uncomfortable for patients with dry eyes or for those who live and work in polluted city air. They may cause visual aberrations (including halos and uneven vision) and always carry an increased risk of infection and possible corneal scarring. Individuals who live in higher altitudes may become intolerant of contact lenses over time because of less oxygen and lower humidity in the air.

The variety of contact lenses available today is dazzling. Costs for contacts vary widely, depending on the type you need.

Orthokeratology

This is a technique for treating myopia, or nearsightedness. *Orthokeratology* uses a series of rigid contact lenses that apply pressure to the sides of the cornea to flatten them. The effects are not permanent and require continued dependence on daily-wear maintenance lenses to retain the reshaping. The technique is expensive, high maintenance, and requires continuous follow-up visits. Long-term effects can include permanently warped corneas. The risk of infection is also greater than that from normal contact lens wear.

2

Laser Vision Correction

People have understood the mechanics of eyesight for thousands of years. Writings and drawings on this subject from the ancient Islamic world go back as far as 2000 B.C. And the quest to correct vision has never stopped. From the invention of eyeglasses hundreds of years ago to the fabrication of the first American contact lenses, the evolution of vision correction has, indeed, been astonishing. Now zoom ahead a few decades to the development of laser surgery, today one of the most popular methods of vision correction. The advent of computers and laser technology has made it possible to perform laser eye surgery to correct the shape of the cornea.

History of Vision Correction Surgery

Although many pioneering contributions lead to the development of modern *refractive surgery* (any surgical procedure to help the eye focus light correctly), one of the key breakthroughs happened in the middle of the last century. In 1949 Dr. José Barraquer of Bogotá, Colombia developed the idea of *lamellar* (layered) *corneal surgery*. Barraquer discovered that lamellar surgery could reshape the cornea, enhancing the eye's ability to focus. To do so, he removed a disc of the front portion of the cornea with an instrument called a *microkeratome*. This instrument is affixed to the eye by using a vacuum ring; then a sharp, thin blade shaves a small amount of the cornea at a predetermined depth. Dr. Barraquer then froze the disc before grinding it into a new shape with a small lathe. He then replaced the newly shaped disc back onto the cornea. The procedure of carving the cornea was called *keratomileusis*.

Two important refinements followed. In 1985, Dr. Casimir Swinger developed a method of reshaping the disc without freezing it (*nonfreeze keratomileusis*). Then in 1987, Dr. Luis Ruiz, a protégé of Barraquer, used an automated microkeratome to reshape the cornea directly on the eye. This procedure, *automated lamellar keratoplasty (ALK)*, was used to correct high levels of myopia and hyperopia. Importantly, patients who have undergone these two procedures, precursors to today's laser vision correction, have not experienced long-term complications from the corneal reshaping.

The Arrival of the Excimer Laser

The *excimer laser* was first used on human eyes in the late 1980s. The laser technology marked a significant advancement in the science of vision correction—the excimer laser uses a cool, ultraviolet beam of light to vaporize tissue with a great deal of precision, without harming adjacent tissue. Each pulse of the excimer laser removes 1/4000 millimeter of tissue by breaking up the molecules that hold this tissue together. It would take about 200 pulses from an excimer laser to cut a human hair in half.

PRK

The first widely used procedure with the excimer laser, *photorefractive keratectomy (PRK)* began in 1987. Instead of using a microkeratome to reshape the cornea, PRK uses the laser to accurately sculpt the cornea one microscopic layer at a time. PRK has vastly improved since those early days.

PRK sculpts the cornea by first removing the epithelium, the outer protective layer of the cornea. The laser works its way down into the stroma, or structural part of the cornea, where the real reshaping takes place. Although the epithelium eventually grows back, the process presents some nagging problems. First, PRK leaves the patient's eyes sore for forty-eight hours after surgery. Second, the corneal surface, left exposed, results in blurred vision for almost a week and has an increased chance of infection. Third, the healing process from the PRK may produce *corneal haze*, a clouding in the cornea caused by the healing process; this can blur the vision and can alter the accuracy of the treatment. (See appendix.)

LASIK

In 1991, researchers conceived of ways to avoid these problems with a new procedure called LASIK. The components of LASIK are defined as:

Laser—performed with the excimer laser

In situ—the cornea in its natural position on the eye

Keratomileusis—a process of carving the cornea to reshape it

With LASIK, the cornea—rather than being surgically removed, reshaped, and then reattached—is sculpted right on the eye using the excimer laser as the sculpting tool. An extremely thin flap of the outer layer of the cornea is created using a state-of-the-art microkeratome. The flap, like a clear, hinged lid, is gently lifted back, exposing the stroma beneath. After the surgeon sculpts the stroma to correct its shape, the flap is set back in place. Amazingly, the flap is held in position by the eye's natural suction, providing increased comfort and decreased recovery time for the patient.

Layers of the Cornea

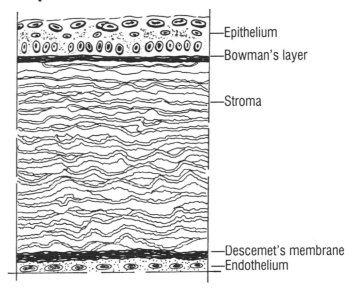

The eyeball cornea, about as thick as a credit card, is made up of many layers. When LASIK is performed, surgeons reshape the stroma layer, changing the way light bends as it enters the eye.

Clinical trials on LASIK began in the United States in 1996. A broad series of clinical investigations culminated in its approval by the FDA in 1999.

LASIK offers numerous advantages over PRK and has become the surgery of choice for both doctors and patients.

PRK and LASIK: A Comparison

	PRK	**LASIK**
Range of correction	Low to moderate	Low to severe
Depth of penetration	Superficial	20 percent
Intraoperative pain	Minimal	Minimal
Postoperative pain	Moderate, 24-48 hours	Minimal, 12 hours
Postoperative medications	1-3 months, possibly longer	1 week
Functional vision recovery	3-5 days	24 hours
Visual results fully recognized	3 weeks to several months	1-4 weeks
Return to work	3-5 days	1 day
Risk of complications	Low (less surgeon dependent)	Low (more surgeon dependent
Risk of haze (scarring) in the central cornea	1-2 percent	Less than 1 percent

How LASIK Corrects the Eye's Focus

How can a laser beam correct vision? The excimer laser is uniquely suited to the task of refractive corneal surgery because it *ablates*, or vaporizes, tissue by breaking apart the molecules without creating damaging heat. The unparalleled precision of the excimer laser makes it the ultimate reshaping tool. Each pulse of the laser removes the equivalent of 1/2000 of a human hair in 4 billionths of a second. This allows the surgeon to sculpt the exposed corneal bed, gently and precisely, into a more desirable shape that allows rays of light to focus properly on the retina.

LASIK and Myopic Correction

As explained earlier, patients who are nearsighted have corneas with too much curvature in proportion to the length of their eyes. Once the corneal flap is made and lifted back, the excimer laser reshapes the underlying stroma to achieve a flatter cornea. The surgeon's careful, precise measurements, programmed into the computer, guide the excimer laser. When the reshaping is complete, the flap is replaced. The result is that light rays coming through the cornea now come to a point of focus on the retina, rather than in front of it.

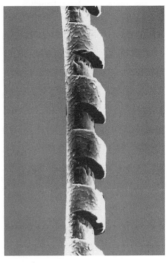

This human hair, which has been ablated by an excimer laser, shows the precision with which the laser works. *Photo courtesy of VISX.*

LASIK and Hyperopic Correction

Farsighted patients, on the other hand, have corneas that are proportionately too flat for the length of their eyes. The excimer laser is programmed to remove tissue from just the periphery of the stroma, leaving the middle untouched; this creates more of a domed shape. The increased curvature of the cornea will allow light rays to focus on the retina, rather than behind it.

LASIK and Astigmatism

To treat astigmatism, the excimer laser removes tissue in a somewhat oval fashion, adjusting the shape of the cornea in one axis more than the other. The goal is to produce a symmetrical surface so that light rays passing through the cornea at various places will all meet at a single point of focus on the retina.

LASIK: State of the Art

No LASIK surgeon can promise 20/20 vision without the use of corrective eyeglasses or contact lenses. However, better than 99 percent of typical myopic patients after LASIK can clearly read the two or three lines of letters adjacent to the 20/20 line of the Snellen eye chart without the help of eyeglasses or contacts. In fact, the vast majority of patients can drive without glasses (for which 20/40 vision is required) the day after LASIK surgery.

3

Contemplating Laser Eye Surgery

I f you have worn eyeglasses or contacts most of your life, the possibility of having good eyesight without them may have seemed remote. But today, high success rates with LASIK are inspiring more people to seriously contemplate laser eye surgery. A good way to get started is to address these two questions: (1) Am I a good candidate for LASIK? and (2) How do I find the best surgeon?

Am I a Good Candidate for LASIK?

Whether LASIK is the best option for you will ultimately depend on the judgment of your eye surgeon, who makes that determination during a preoperative evaluation. However, good candidates for LASIK have some basic conditions in common.

Ideal Age

A good candidate is at least eighteen years old, since the vision of people younger than eighteen often continues to change. Myopia may continue to increase in some patients until their mid- to late twenties.

Stable Prescription

No matter what your age, to be considered a good candidate for LASIK you need to have a stable prescription, which means your prescription should not have changed more than 1 diopter a year.

Treatable Eyesight Parameters

Good candidates for LASIK have refractive errors that fall within certain parameters. If you are nearsighted, you may have myopia of –0.75 to –12.00 diopters. If farsighted, your hyperopia may be up to +6.00 diopters. Your level of astigmatism may be as high as 6.00 diopters. These are normal parameters, but they can vary from patient to patient and from doctor to doctor, depending on the type of excimer laser used.

Surgically Ideal Eyes

You will not know until the preoperative examination whether your eyes meet the standards required for LASIK. These would include:

- A correctly sized pupil (not too large)
- A cornea of the right thickness (not too thin)
- A cornea that is structurally normal (not irregularly shaped)
- Healthy pressure within the eye
- Generally healthy eyes (no eye diseases or injuries that could interfere)

Conditions That May Prevent Surgery

Any number of factors could make you a poor candidate for LASIK. Some patients fear their eyesight is too poor, yet later discover, after meeting with their eye doctor, that it falls within treatable parameters that yield successful outcomes. So, do not assume you are a poor candidate until you have consulted with your ophthalmologist and he or she confirms it.

Unstable Prescription

You should not contemplate LASIK if you are under eighteen, or if your eye prescription changes regularly or has changed by more than 1 diopter in the past twelve months.

Severe Refractive Error

If your refractive error is so severe that it falls outside normal treatable parameters, you may not be an ideal candidate for LASIK. To correct extreme nearsightedness or farsightedness requires too much deep sculpting and corneal reshaping. Other vision correction procedures may be preferable. But to be certain, get your eye doctor's opinion.

Some people aren't good candidates for LASIK. When I recommend against the surgery, my concern is that these patients will go somewhere else and have the surgery done when they shouldn't.

Dr. Robert Maloney

Other Health Conditions

You may be a poor candidate for LASIK if you have any of the following conditions:

- *Atypically large pupils.* If a pupil is wider than the laser beam, the area outside the beam will not be shaped by the laser. After surgery, the patient will see through the "old," untreated area as well as the newly treated area. Complications may include poor night vision, ghosting of images, and star bursts associated with dim light conditions.

- *Thin cornea.* A thin cornea will not retain its structure and shape if the top layers of tissue are surgically removed.

- *Abnormally structured cornea.* This condition is not treatable with LASIK.

- *Pregnant or nursing.* These conditions might change the measured refraction in the eye.

- *Collagen vascular disease.* These diseases affect the collagen-containing connective tissue.

- *Glaucoma or cataracts.* These active eye diseases may cause complications for laser surgery. Glaucoma is a disorder of the eye characterized by an increase of pressure within the eyeball; cataracts are a clouding of the lens within the eye causing decreased vision.

- Certain *corneal dystrophies.* These conditions are usually inherited conditions in which one or more parts of the cornea lose normal clarity due to a buildup of cloudy material.

- Active *herpetic keratitis,* a herpes infection in the eye.

- *Diabetic retinopathy.* This is a potentially blinding complication of diabetes that damages the eye's retina.

- *Heart disease.* Heart conditions that require use of a pacemaker.

Some conditions such as lupus, rheumatoid arthritis, and diabetes may not exclude you from having LASIK vision correction, but these conditions must by controlled and identified. Discuss the suitability for the procedure with your surgeon if you have any of the above conditions.

Prescription Medicines That May Cause Problems

You are not a good candidate for LASIK if you are taking certain prescription medications, including:

- *Accutane*, prescribed to treat severe acne. This drug may cause severe dry eyes and decreased night vision.

- Oral *prednisone*, most commonly prescribed for severe allergies, asthma, or arthritis. This drug may lower your resistance to infections.

Your ophthalmologist will ask you about all prescription and over-the-counter medications you are taking and how long you have been on them.

Unrealistic Expectations

Unrealistic expectations are a risk in the sense that the patient will almost certainly be disappointed with the outcome of laser eye surgery. As a patient, it is your responsibility to understand exactly what the procedure can and cannot do. For example, you might still need eyeglasses for performing certain activities, such as viewing a subtitled film or driving at night. It is best to think of LASIK as reducing your dependence on eyeglasses and contact lenses and improving your natural vision.

Usually, LASIK will correct your distance vision permanently. However, eyesight changes slightly over time, from one year to the next. In the years following LASIK, your eyes may still change slightly, not because the procedure was unstable, but because our eyes change. It this occurs, a LASIK *enhancement procedure* can be performed even many years later.

An enhancement procedure is a retreatment with the laser, usually at least three to six months following the original LASIK surgery; this procedure fine-tunes the shape of the cornea after the patient's vision has stabilized. Enhancements are a normal part of LASIK, even in the hands of the most skilled and experienced surgeon. Each person's tissue responds differently to the excimer laser, both during the surgery and while healing; as a result, 5 to 10 percent of patients need enhancements.

The most important thing is that a patient's expectations be met. The only way for a doctor to do that is to spend time with a patient and learn about why he or she wants the procedure and what the patient's goals are.

Dr. Ernest Kornmehl

Finding the Right LASIK Surgeon

If you are a good candidate for LASIK, your next step will be the most important one: finding the right physician to perform the procedure. You will need an *ophthalmologist* to perform your LASIK surgery. An ophthalmologist is a licensed medical doctor who has a minimum of four years of additional training after medical school. This advanced training usually involves a one-year internship in internal medicine or general surgery, followed by three to four years in an ophthalmology residency. A select group of ophthalmologists completes an additional year or two of fellowship training in corneal surgery.

Ask for Referrals

If you know people who have had the LASIK procedure, ask them who their surgeon was and how they felt about their overall experience. Were they happy with the outcome? Did they have confidence in their surgeon? Was the surgeon compassionate, and did he or she take time to answer questions before and after the procedure? Was the support staff helpful? Personal experiences are powerful indicators of the quality of care.

Ask Your Optometrist or Ophthalmologist

An eye care practitioner whom you trust and respect is another good source of referrals. Since referring patients is a routine and important part of their professional practice, these physicians will almost always be able to recommend ophthalmologists near you who are experienced with LASIK and have sound reputations.

Contact Ophthalmic Boards and Medical Associations

Some medical organizations, such as the American Board of Ophthalmology, provide information about physicians free of charge to consumers. Ask for names of ophthalmologists who specialize in corneal and refractive surgery who have been certified by the board. The American Academy of Ophthalmology also has a web site, www.eyenet.org, where you may search for board-certified eye doctors by city, state, and specialty (refractive surgery). The site lists doctor's practice focus, current professional activity, educational history and degrees, residency, fellowships, teaching positions, certification, contact information, and often a web site address. More information on how to contact this organization is listed in the Resource section in the back of this book.

The International Society of Refractive Surgery also maintains a list of member surgeons on its web site, www.isrs.org. The list is organized by city and state. Note that membership in this and other organizations does not necessarily mean the surgeon is board certified.

Check your local library for The American Board of Medical Specialties' four-volume *Official ABMS Directory of Board Certified Medical Specialists.* This publication lists refractive surgeons by region who have been certified by the American Board of Ophthalmology. To verify whether a specific eye doctor is board certified, you can also call ABMS at 866–ASK–ABMS (275–2267).

Using the Internet

If you like doing consumer research on the Internet, you will find much information about LASIK on-line. Keep in mind, however, that the Internet is an unsupervised and largely unregulated media. There is no guarantee that the information you get on the Internet will be either accurate or complete.

You may also find directories, both on-line and off line, that list surgeons who perform LASIK. Some physician directories are not exhaustive listings of all refractive surgeons practicing in your area. Rather, they may comprise physicians who have chosen to be listed, often for a fee. Since the majority of these sites do not check a surgeon's credentials, be sure to research the doctor's credentials thoroughly.

Questions to Ask About a Surgeon

Once you have the names of refractive surgeons, the next step is to find out more about their credentials, reputation, and practice. LASIK surgeons understand and appreciate that patients will have many questions about them and about the procedure. When you find a doctor with promising credentials, call the office and ask to speak with the LASIK coordinator or a staff member who can answer patient's questions. If you feel it's necessary to meet with the surgeon directly, understand that the surgeon's time is valuable, and you will likely be charged for the consultation.

What Are the Surgeon's Credentials?

Consider only surgeons who are board certified. What does this mean? In addition to the medical education, internship and residency program mentioned earlier, ophthalmologists must pass a series of exams given by the National Board of Medical Examiners; they must also pass two additional examinations administered by the American Board of Ophthalmology. After passing these final exams, physicians are certified by the American Board of Ophthalmology.

Some ophthalmologists are *fellowship trained* cornea or refractive surgeons. This means they have been offered one or two years of extra training in diseases and surgery of the cornea under the supervision of leading physicians in the field. These fellowship-trained surgeons will likely have a lower incidence of complications because they can diagnose subtle findings prior to surgery.

Surgeons may attain training and further certification by the American College of Surgeons, known for its steep credentialing process. Once a member, or fellow, the physician becomes a Fellow of the American College of Surgeons, and the initials F.A.C.S., will be listed after his or her name.

How Many LASIK Procedures Has the Surgeon Performed?

Be specific in asking about a physician's experience with LASIK, since other laser procedures require different skills than those required for LASIK. Because there is a learning curve, surgeons should have performed a minimum of 1,000 LASIK procedures; research shows that the complication rate for surgeons is reduced even further after they have performed 3,000 procedures.

It generally takes 1,000 LASIK procedures before a surgeon's *nomogram* is reasonably well developed. The nomogram refers to the formula the surgeon enters into the excimer laser computer for each procedure. Even though excimer lasers come from the manufacturer with recommended settings to correct the various refractive errors, the surgeon fine-tunes and customizes these settings with the nomogram. Based on a series of measurements the surgeon takes during the preoperative exam, the nomogram includes factors such as the degree of refractive error and the patient's age. It also takes into consideration the surgeon's own technique and the type of laser he or she will use. A well-developed and artful nomogram allows the surgeon to more accurately program the laser for each patient, decreasing the probability that an enhancement procedure will be necessary.

The three most important qualities in a surgeon are: obsessive attention to detail, statistical sophistication in analyzing surgery results, and having a lot of experience.

Dr. Robert Maloney

How Many Procedures Has the Surgeon Performed on Patients with Your Refractive Error?

Perhaps as important as the total number of LASIK procedures a surgeon has completed is the number he or she has performed on patients with the same refractive error as yours using the same laser equipment. The surgeon should have completed 100 or more such procedures. Even an experienced surgeon could have difficulty with certain less common refractive errors. And new equipment takes some getting used to as well. Additionally, the surgeon should have experience with patients of your age, gender, and race—relevant because the surgical techniques needed to correct refractive errors in these groups may differ slightly.

Ask to Speak with Former Patients

Ask a prospective surgeon for the names of two or three patients you can contact who had a refractive error similar to your own. This is not an unusual request. When you speak with them, ask how they felt about the surgeon, the staff, and the quality of their LASIK experience.

How Does the Surgeon Track LASIK Procedure Outcomes?

The surgeon's response to this question will reveal much. If the surgeon has readily available statistics in the form of charts and graphs, he or she is most likely *benchmarking,* or tracking, LASIK outcomes. In addition, if the surgeon presents his or her data at well-respected national or international conferences to other surgeons, or publishes in professional journals, you can be confident that he or she is tracking outcomes.

Benchmarking is very important because it indicates the surgeon is concerned about achieving the best possible results over time. There is no mandatory central reporting database for tracking LASIK outcomes, unless a surgeon is participating in a sanctioned clinical trial. Therefore, doing so voluntarily indicates high personal standards of professionalism and performance.

In tracking data, it is important that your surgeon has performed a statistically significant number of procedures. With data from 1,000 or more procedures, your surgeon would be able to predict outcomes fairly accurately.

What Are the Surgeon's Success and Complication Rates?

The physician or the LASIK coordinator should be able to give you the percentage of LASIK patients whose procedures result in 20/40 vision or better. It's normal for more than 95 percent of LASIK patients to achieve this level of vision. Ask what percentage of the physician's LASIK patients receive 20/20 vision. Your surgeon should be able to tell you based on 1,000 or more procedures and your level of refractive error. Ask what percentage of LASIK patients report significant complications. Less than 1 percent is acceptable. Keep in mind that most complications, if they do occur, can be managed by an experienced surgeon.

Has the Surgeon Participated in Research Activities, Lecturing, or Writing?

Doctors who have researched and written articles for peer-reviewed journals, been speakers at medical conferences, and/or published books are usually well respected among their peers. This is an indication of the physician's experience and competence. This level of professional involvement, above and beyond his or her ophthalmology practice, shows the doctor's mastery, motivation, and passion in the field.

Has the Surgeon Ever Been Asked to Participate in an FDA Clinical Trial?

The Food and Drug Administration (FDA) invites some ophthalmologists to participate as principal investigators in *clinical trials* sanctioned by laser manufacturers. A clinical trial is a research study, conducted with patients, that is designed to evaluate the safety and effectiveness of a new procedure or device. Typically, FDA-selected ophthalmologists are chosen because of their demonstrated skill and ability, and their complete understanding of laser vision correction and the laser being used. These surgeons are subject to detailed analysis and reporting, and are willing to endure extreme scrutiny.

Note that an ophthalmologist may be very competent to perform LASIK but has never been asked to participate in a clinical trial. Still, if you've found a surgeon who has participated in a clinical trial, you've likely found one of the best.

Has the Doctor Ever Been Sued for Malpractice?

Even the best surgeon may have had a malpractice suit brought against him or her, so be careful about passing judgment based on what might have been a frivolous lawsuit. But multiple lawsuits against a doctor would require an explanation. More than one lawsuit for every decade of practice is a bad sign. If you are embarrassed to ask about malpractice suits against the doctor, there are alternate ways to obtain this information.

One organization, the Association of State Medical Board Executive Directors, is a group of participating state licensing authorities that provides malpractice and disciplinary action information about specific doctors. The Association's information is free and available at their web site www.docboard.org. However, not every state in the nation participates.

The Federation of State Medical Boards is another organization that collects and disseminates information about doctors' malpractice histories. The charge is $9.95 for each request, and it takes five to seven days to get the answer. Contact the organization at their web site, www.fsmb.org, or write to them at the address listed in the Resource section.

Finally, on-line services provide background information on every physician licensed to practice medicine in the United States. One such service, Medi-Net, includes nationwide records of any sanctions or disciplinary actions taken against a physician, plus his or her state license, board certification, education, residencies, and specialties. The on-line fee for this information is $14.95 per name. The web site is www.searchpointe.com.

How Many Patients Does the Surgeon Turn Away?

A conscientious surgeon might turn away as many as 15 to 20 percent of the patients he or she evaluates during the preoperative examination. Be wary of a doctor who rarely advises a patient against the procedure. Many factors can make a patient a poor candidate for LASIK. No doctor with high ethical standards will perform laser surgery on your eyes if you are not a good candidate.

Will the Doctor Be Personally Involved in My Preoperative and Postoperative Care?

Avoid the "shopping mall" approach to surgery, where patients are shuffled through to the surgical suite without having first met with the surgeon. Most doctors have knowledgeable and compassionate staff to help perform tests and answer questions. However, it is also important to have met with the surgeon before signing any documents, saying you agree to have the surgery.

The style of care that makes you feel comfortable is something only you can determine. Ask the LASIK coordinator if the surgeon will be conducting the preoperative exam.

Some patients choose to see their regular optometrist or ophthalmologist for their preoperative and postoperative care. If you plan to do this, be sure your surgeon is comfortable working with your primary eye doctor. While the majority of people have an uncomplicated postoperative course, you want to make sure your care provider will be able to recognize complications if they arise, and can either treat you or refer you for treatment before more serious, long-term repercussions occur.

What Type of Laser Does the Surgeon Use?

Make sure your doctor uses an FDA-approved excimer laser. Laser technology has improved dramatically over the past five years. The state of the art lasers now have eye tracking, which further improves the safety of the procedure. For example, if your eye moves accidentally during the treatment, the laser will automatically follow it. Ask your surgeon if he or she uses an eye tracking laser.

These state-of-the-art lasers also allow larger diameter treatment areas, which minimizes the risk of nighttime glare.

The FDA web site, www.fda.gov, also has links to laser manufacturers' web sites, where some maintain lists of doctors certified to use their machines. If your doctor is not listed, you may wish to contact the laser manufacturer directly. Verify that the doctor has been certified by the laser company to operate a particular machine, which means he or she took a required training course.

How Much Does LASIK Cost?

Cost should not be the main factor in choosing a LASIK surgeon. First and foremost, seek out a surgeon who has a good reputation in the medical community and plenty of experience. If you are swayed by low cost, this may signal trouble for you down the road. Find the best-qualified surgeon with high medical standards for patient care, compassionate staff to tend to your needs, comprehensive postoperative care, enhancement procedures if necessary, and availability if any problems or complications crop up after surgery.

The cost of LASIK varies from surgeon to surgeon. Generally, LASIK runs between $1,500 and $3,000 per eye. Be sure to ask whether preoperative and postoperative care as well as enhancement procedures are included in the quoted per-eye cost.

Making the Decision

Sometimes, no matter how much information you have gathered, the decision to go with one surgeon over another comes down to feelings. Personal chemistry is extremely important. Choose someone with whom you feel comfortable—someone who is easy to talk to, friendly, and professional. Naturally, you also want a surgeon who listens to your questions, answers them completely, and asks you questions as well. A good doctor-patient relationship is important in devising a treatment plan that best suits your needs. Likewise, the surgeon's support staff should be highly trained, competent, and caring. These are the people who will help support you through the LASIK procedure.

Once you feel comfortable with your decision after carefully researching surgeons in your area, you're probably ready to schedule your initial consultation.

4

The Consultation

Your initial consultation, prior to a procedure, is your opportunity to get to know the surgeon and to ask as many questions as necessary in order to feel safe and comfortable undergoing LASIK. Many patients prefer to invite a friend, spouse, or other family member to sit in on the meeting with the surgeon. Taking someone along may be helpful. He or she may help you remember questions to ask, or may help you recall information later.

The consultation is also the surgeon's chance to get to know you, to gain an understanding of your expectations, and to do an initial examination of your eyes. At the end of the consultation, the surgeon should be able to tell whether you are a good candidate for LASIK and what your outcome will likely be.

The Initial Appointment

A preoperative consultation usually takes about an hour and a half. When you call to make an appointment, you will be asked about the type of contact lenses you wear, if any. You'll also be given instructions about your contacts in preparation for the consultation.

- If you wear soft, spherical contact lenses, you will need to stop wearing them forty-eight hours to one week before your consultation.

- If you wear *toric* contact lenses, you may need to stop wearing them forty-eight hours to one week before your consultation. Toric lenses are soft lenses designed for astigmatism. They are slightly oval shaped and are weighted so they will not rotate on the eye.

- If you wear hard contact lenses, *rigid gas permeable (RGP)* lenses, you may need to stop wearing them at least two weeks before your consultation. RGP lenses are made of a porous substance that permits oxygen to permeate the lenses so the eyes can "breathe."

Why discontinue wearing contact lenses prior to the eye exam? Contact lenses can alter the shape of your cornea for up to several weeks after you have stopped wearing them, depending on the type of lens. For the surgeon to take accurate measurements, the cornea must assume its natural shape. Your surgeon may need to repeat these measurements after your initial consultation and before surgery to make sure the shape of your cornea has stabilized.

Your Medical and Vision History

When meeting with your surgeon for the first time, he or she will want to get a sense of your overall health and the health of your eyes. It is important for your surgeon to know everything about your medical history. Some systemic diseases like rheumatoid arthritis and lupus, certain healing disorders, diabetes, and a current or planned pregnancy demand special consideration when it comes to laser vision correction.

Your surgeon must be made aware of any history of *herpes simplex* on the eye. This disease is a recurrent viral infection characterized by a painful sore on the eyelid or surface of the eye; it causes inflammation of the cornea and can lead to blindness. Although this condition would not necessarily disqualify you from having LASIK altogether, an active viral outbreak would require that the surgery be postponed until the eyeball is completely healed, with no recurrence for at least six months. Genital herpes simplex or cold sores on your lips do not create a problem for LASIK surgery.

Also tell your surgeon about any ongoing changes or problems you have had with your vision. For example, if you have a significant cataract or experience the symptoms associated with cataracts, you should not undergo LASIK vision correction. Such symptoms include glare from lamps or very bright light, frequent changes in your eyeglass prescription, and cloudy or blurred vision.

Be sure to tell your surgeon about any problems you've had with contact lenses, or any other eye-related discomfort you have been having, no matter how trivial it seems. For example, patients often turn to laser eye surgery when their contacts have become too uncomfortable to wear because of dry eyes.

The Medical Examination

The next part of the preoperative consultation involves a series of eye tests and evaluations that provide the necessary data before a LASIK procedure. These may be conducted at your surgeon's office or by your regular eye doctor.

In either case, the physician will measure your refractive error and determine which of your eyes is dominant. Next, he/she will measure your cornea with a *corneal topographer,* an instrument that uses computerized analysis to arrive at an extremely accurate three-dimensional "map" of your cornea. This test will reveal whether you have a structurally abnormal cornea, which could disqualify you as a candidate for LASIK.

The thickness of your cornea will be measured with a *pachymeter.* Because a certain amount of tissue will be surgically removed, or ablated, during the LASIK procedure, your cornea must be thick enough for the remaining tissue to retain its structure and shape. If your cornea is too thin, you would not be a good LASIK candidate.

Next, the size of your pupil will be measured. The diameter of the *ablation zone,* or the area in which tissue will be removed by the laser, should be greater than the diameter of your pupil when it is dilated, or wide open, as under low-light conditions. If your pupil is too large, you could experience glare, light sensitivity, or other symptoms. As emphasized earlier, individuals with atypically large pupils are not ideal candidates for LASIK.

Your eyes will also be examined with a special scope so that the cornea can be studied in microscopic detail. The doctor will be checking for abnormalities at the cellular level that could be symptomatic of eye disease.

Then he or she will measure the *intraocular pressure* of your eyes, also called *tonometry.* This tests the pressure exerted by the fluid (vitreous humor) within the eyeball that gives it a round, firm shape. Increased pressure could be an indication of glaucoma.

Next, drops will be put in your eyes. These drops temporarily relax focusing muscles, dilating the pupil. Your refractive error will again be measured and the doctor will examine the back of the eye, including the retina and the optic nerve. In nearsighted patients these dilating eyedrops will not affect distance vision, which is needed for driving, but will blur near vision for about four to six hours.

Questions to Ask About LASIK

LASIK surgeons are accustomed to having patients ask questions. Part of the physician's role is to educate you as thoroughly as possible. Many LASIK centers offer written material designed to address your questions. Other LASIK centers show short videos that explain the procedure in detail. However, if you still have questions, or just want to discuss any reservations or fears, the consultation is the best time to do it.

For most patients, the more they know, the more comfortable they are. For other patients, the less they know, the more comfortable they are. Still, every patient needs to be informed.

Dr. Jonathan Davidorf

Is LASIK Painful?

No. Before the procedure begins, your eye is numbed with eyedrops. You may feel a slight sensation of pressure as the corneal flap is being made, but actual pain is rare. After the surgery, any discomfort you experience will last only a few hours. Sleep and lubricating eyedrops, as well as Tylenol or ibuprofen, are usually enough to take care of any discomfort.

How Long Does LASIK Take?

Most patients are pleasantly surprised at how quickly LASIK is performed. Expect LASIK to take between five to ten minutes for each eye.

How Long Will It Take for My Eyes to Heal?

Compared to other laser eye surgeries, the normal healing process is fast, with fewer associated side effects. Most postoperative discomfort and visual side effects are quite minor. You may notice a burning sensation and may experience watery eyes in one or both eyes for a few hours after surgery, but usually by the very next day you should not have any significant eye discomfort. The most common discomfort that sometimes persists is dry eye. Symptoms related to post-LASIK dry eye are usually minor, can be alleviated with lubricating eyedrops, and generally disappear within two to six months. In terms of visual acuity, most patients notice good vision the day after surgery. Visual clarity and crispness after LASIK tends to improve for two to six months before stabilizing.

What Results Can I Expect?

Results vary. Finding a skilled and experienced surgeon maximizes your chances for the best possible outcome. However, with higher degrees of myopia, hyperopia, and astigmatism, results are less predictable and enhancement procedures are more common.

How Long Will the Correction Last?

Once your eye has stabilized, usually in two to three months, your correction is permanent. If you eventually need eyeglasses for reading after that, it would be the result of the normal aging process.

What About Risks and Complications?

It is not unusual for people considering LASIK to experience fear, nervousness, and uncertainty at first. Most patients feel a lot better about the procedure once they become fully informed. Knowing the statistical improbability of a serious complication goes a long way toward relieving your fears.

Your doctor should inform you about the risks and potential complications associated with LASIK, ranging from very minor, short-term discomfort to serious complications, which are rare. He or she should also explain what you can do to avoid some of these risks. Fortunately, the incidence of serious complications is low in the hands of a skilled and experienced surgeon. More details about risks and possible complications appear in chapter 8.

Will I Be Able to Drive Immediately After LASIK?

No, you should not drive upon leaving the clinic. You will need a driver. But with LASIK you can usually drive the very next day, and almost certainly within two days. State departments of motor vehicles typically grant unrestricted driving privileges to people with 20/40 or better vision. Over 90 percent of all patients who undergo LASIK have this level of vision or better the day after surgery.

When Can I Go Back to Work?

Most patients can return to work the day after their LASIK procedure. If you work in a very dusty environment, such as a construction site, wait forty-eight hours before going back to work.

Although most patients can function normally at work the day after surgery, it is recommended that you not schedule any unbreakable appointments or meetings for that day.

Will I Need Enhancement Surgery?

If an eye is undercorrected or overcorrected with LASIK, you can undergo an enhancement procedure. But first your eye must stabilize, which usually takes two to three months after the original surgery.

With an enhancement procedure, the corneal flap will not need to be recreated. Instead, the surgeon, using a specialized instrument, gently lifts the preexisting flap and performs the additional laser treatment. Recovery time is similar to the original procedure. You may or may not be charged an additional fee for such enhancement surgery.

If I Have Dry Eyes, Will It Affect My LASIK Surgery?

Many patients consider LASIK because they have dry eyes and cannot wear contact lenses. If you have dry eyes, it is important that they be treated before surgery. Tear supplements and *punctum plugs* (tiny silicone plugs placed in the tear drainage openings of your eyelid) should keep them moist.

After LASIK, your eyes may feel drier. This condition is temporary, typically lasting one week to six months. Dry-eye symptoms can be particularly noticeable if you use a computer frequently, read for long periods of time, or drive extended distances. For many patients, it is useful to use lubricating eyedrops often, especially for the first few weeks after surgery.

If I've Had Previous Eye Surgeries, Am I Still a Candidate for LASIK?

Patients who have had certain types of eye surgery are sometimes candidates for LASIK as a second procedure to improve their vision. However, these are often more difficult surgeries with less predictable results.

For example, LASIK has been used following an older form of refractive surgery, *radial keratotomy (RK)*. With RK, the cornea is flattened by making small, spokelike incisions around its periphery to correct myopia and astigmatism. LASIK following RK can succeed as long as the patient's vision is relatively stable and there is not significant corneal scarring.

Follow-up care is important, too. I encourage patients to ask a lot of questions about the quality of follow-up care they'll receive after a LASIK procedure.

Dr. Jonathan Davidorf

Patients who have had a corneal transplant can have a LASIK procedure to enhance results. This is especially effective for those who develop a high degree of astigmatism caused by the surgery. A clear corneal transplant will allow good vision only if it has a relatively round surface. Laser vision correction can smooth out astigmatic curves in the cornea.

Can I Wear Contact Lenses After Surgery, If Necessary?

After surgery, if you still need correction in one or both eyes and choose not to have an enhancement procedure, you may elect to wear contact lenses. With LASIK, you may wear contacts within a few weeks. If you had no previous problems with contacts before LASIK, it is doubtful you will have problems afterward.

Could the Surgery Cause Problems Years from Now?

The chance of problems years down the road is very unlikely. LASIK is a form of lamellar refractive surgery, a type of surgery that has been performed since 1949. Importantly, patients who have undergone earlier types of lamellar refractive surgery—much less accurate and more invasive than LASIK—have not developed any unusual problems during the past fifty years.

Will Having LASIK Prevent Other Eye Diseases?

No. LASIK does not prevent cataracts, glaucoma, retinal detachment, macular degeneration, or any other eye disease. Ophthalmologists refer to LASIK as *disease neutral.* That is, LASIK does not prevent diseases, and if you are diagnosed with a disease in the future, LASIK will not affect its treatment.

Are There New Developments I Should Know About?

Most doctors keep up with the latest technology and research in their field. Some attend conferences and lectures. Others immerse themselves in a lifestyle that includes lecturing, writing journal articles, and textbooks, participating in clinical trials for new technology, and consulting for ophthalmology companies. Find out if there's any news that might impact your decision to have LASIK surgery.

Discussing Your Options

After you've had a chance to ask questions, your doctor will discuss with you some options for proceeding with LASIK. There are basically three options: (1) having both eyes done at once, (2) having the eyes done on separate days, and (3) having one eye corrected for close-up vision, and the other eye corrected for distance (monovision).

Although it is optional, most patients prefer to have both eyes done at once. Alternatively, some surgeons as well as patients prefer to treat one eye at a time to reduce risk. Studies have shown, however, that there is no statistically significant difference in accuracy between the two approaches.

Monovision

You may wish to discuss *monovision* with your surgeon if you are in your forties or older. As mentioned earlier, patients approaching middle age begin to develop presbyopia, or difficulty with their fine (close-up) focusing. Patients over the age of forty who have both eyes corrected for distance with LASIK will still eventually need reading glasses to see nearby objects.

Monovision addresses this issue. With monovision, the surgeon corrects your dominant eye for seeing at a distance and your nondominant eye for near vision, thereby reducing the need for reading glasses. When both eyes are functioning together, the brain naturally selects the image from the eye that has the clearer focus. Having eyes for different purposes might sound unsettling, but many patients do quite well with monovision.

Disadvantages include some loss of depth perception and the possibility of impaired night vision. Monovision may not be a good option for certain professions—airplane pilot, bus driver, or professional athlete, for example. Some people also find monovision difficult to get used to. Discuss it with your doctor. He or she may be able to show you with contact lenses what monovision would feel like before you have to make a firm decision.

If you do try monovision and do not like it, you can have an additional laser correction to make the vision in both eyes equal. Ideally, though, it would be better to make this decision beforehand to avoid an additional procedure.

Some surgeons slightly undercorrect the nondominant eye in all patients, so they will always be able to see such things as their watch and a price tag when they enter their mid-forties.

Informed Consent

Based on the examination, if your doctor determines that you are a good candidate for LASIK, he or she will ask you to sign an informed consent form. This is your written legal consent to have the surgeon proceed with your LASIK surgery. Review it carefully, and sign it only after you understand everything on the form. Don't be shy about asking questions.

5

Undergoing LASIK

On the day of your LASIK procedure, it is natural to experience both excitement and nervousness. Patients who feel most at ease on that day are those who have asked questions, read about the LASIK procedure, and perhaps talked with former patients. Understanding LASIK and trusting your surgeon are important to helping you feel confident, calm, and prepared on the day of your procedure.

You won't be able to drive immediately after the procedure, so it is recommended that you have someone drive you to the surgery center and pick you up when you're ready to leave.

Arriving at the Center

Make an effort to arrive at the center rested and relaxed. You should plan to spend one-and-a-half to three hours at the laser center, although this amount of time varies from center to center.

Wear comfortable clothing the day of your surgery. Do not wear makeup, skin moisturizer, perfume, or cologne, since LASIK requires clean, sterile conditions. Earrings should not be worn.

How the LASIK Procedure Is Performed

LASIK is performed while the patient is awake. However, if you are experiencing anxiety, the surgeon may give you a mild oral sedative. Many surgeons talk to the patient throughout the procedure, so the individual knows what is happening and what to expect next.

Before the Procedure

Before the surgery begins, your face will be cleaned with a disinfectant, and you will be asked to wear a surgical cap. You will be given an antibiotic eyedrop and possibly an anti-inflammatory eyedrop. These may sting for a few seconds.

Undergoing the Procedure

Once in the laser suite, you will be positioned comfortably on your back, under the excimer laser. Your surgeon will give you anesthetic eyedrops to numb the

If you're in the hands of a competent surgeon, the incidence of serious complications is remote, so it's important that patients are sure they've found a good surgeon.

Dr. Jonathan Davidorf

surface of your eyes. Your eyelashes will be taped out of the way, and an *eyelid speculum* will be placed between your eyelids, to keep you from blinking. The speculum sometimes causes mild pressure or discomfort to your eyelids at first, but with the numbing drops, these sensations dissipate.

The surgeon will make small reference marks on your cornea with water-soluble ink. These marks will serve as positional guides when it is time to realign the corneal flap.

A suction ring is then placed on your eye to hold it in position to maintain pressure within the eye. Keeping the eye

51

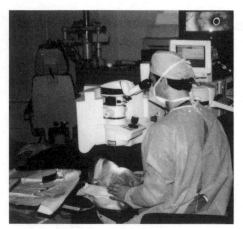

LASIK surgery, being performed here, is done on an outpatient basis.

pressurized is essential for the *keratectomy,* or flap-making process, which comes next. Your vision will dim during this step.

Next the surgeon will create the corneal flap, using the microkeratome, the small instrument with a blade that passes over the eyeball. The extremely thin flap is made from the outermost 25 percent of the cornea. The average cornea, remember, is only about the thickness of a credit card. This flap-making process takes about thirty seconds. When the microkeratome is making the flap, you may feel slight pressure and the instrument will block out light as it passes over your pupil.

Next, the surgeon will ask you to fix your vision on a target light—usually red, green, or yellow. Then, the surgeon will gently lift back the hinged flap. At this point your vision will become blurry.

The surgeon will now perform the laser procedure. This usually takes twenty to ninety seconds. You will not feel any pain as the laser sculpts the cornea by vaporizing small amounts of tissue. This process is called *photoablation*. You will also hear a clicking or buzzing sound with each pulse of the laser. The surgeon is reshaping your cornea.

During the laser procedure, individuals have different responses to staring at the fixation light. Some patients report that the fixation light becomes a blur. Others report that it seems to momentarily disappear. If this happens and your eye starts to wander, the surgeon will stop the laser. You will be coached to look again at the target light so the laser procedure can resume.

Once the process of reshaping your corneal tissue is complete, the excimer laser will be turned off. Using a sterile saline solution, the surgeon will flush the treated surface of the eye to ensure that any debris is washed away. The surgeon then carefully replaces the corneal flap to its original position, using the ink marks as guides.

It takes about one to five minutes for the eye to create a natural vacuum to hold down the flap. The cornea has the unique ability to seal itself back into place. No sutures are necessary. Your eyes will be dried with a sterile cloth, and the eyelid speculum will be removed. You will now be able to blink normally.

At this point, you will be asked to sit with your eyes closed for about thirty minutes. Then your physician will examine your eyes one more time to ensure that the corneal flap is properly positioned.

Patients who have undergone LASIK experience some discomfort, which may last six to eight hours. Patients describe this as a sensation of having sand or a dirty contact lens in their eye. Tylenol, aspirin, ibuprofen, or similar over-the-counter pain medications can help. By the following day, this sensation is usually gone.

Immediately after surgery, expect your vision to be somewhat blurred, similar to looking through a glass of water or wearing a dirty contact lens. However, upon awakening later in the day or the next morning, you should experience improved vision. Most patients report dramatic improvement within twenty-four hours.

Going Home

When you are ready to go home, you will receive antibiotic drops, anti-inflammatory drops to promote healing, and lubricating eye drops, also called "artificial tears." You will be instructed to use these drops frequently. It is common for the eyes to feel somewhat dry after LASIK.

Your surgeon will send you home with detailed instructions on the use of your various eyedrops, and will have given you clear plastic shields to wear at night for the recommended period of time. This is usually from one night to one week. These eye shields prevent accidental trauma to the corneal flap during the healing period, in case you inadvertently bump your eye while you are sleeping.

Your surgeon will probably advise that you go home and take a nap. You may be given a mild sedative to make you sleepy. It is best to have your eyes closed for the first few hours after surgery, and sleep is the easiest way to accomplish this.

LASIK Step-by-Step

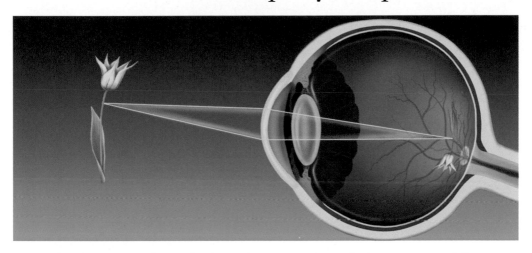

Normal refraction is shown here. Light passes through the cornea and focuses properly on the retina. The result is a clear image of the flower.

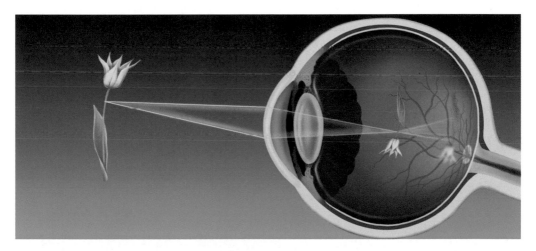

A patient with myopia is represented here. As the flower is viewed, the image is focused in front of the retina, near the middle of the eyeball. As a result, the image that forms on the retina is blurred, as shown by the flower on the right.

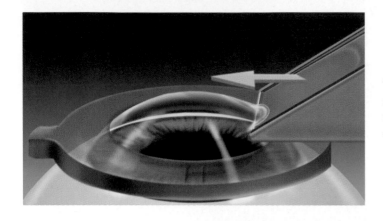

The fine blade of the microkeratome begins to create the thin corneal flap.

The microkeratome continues to advance across the cornea, creating the corneal flap.

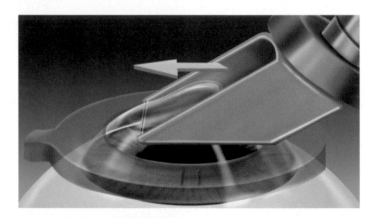

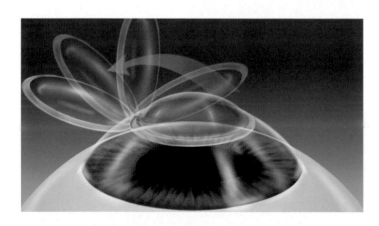

The corneal flap is folded back to expose the bed of the corneal stroma.

The prepared corneal bed is now ready for treatment with the excimer laser.

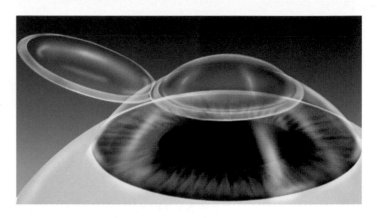

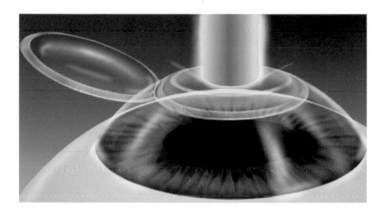

The cool laser beam ablates and reshapes the cornea.

Configuration of the cornea after laser treatment. The laser was preprogrammed to reduce (flatten) the curvature of the cornea.

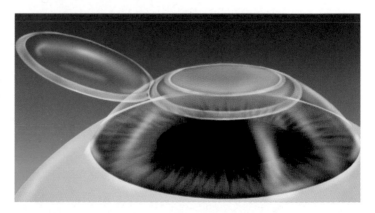

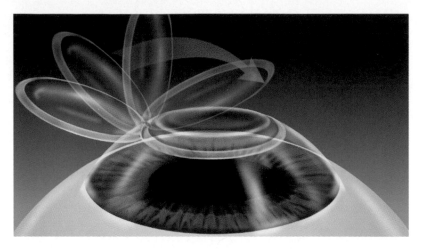

The corneal flap is replaced over the treated corneal stroma.
No sutures are required.

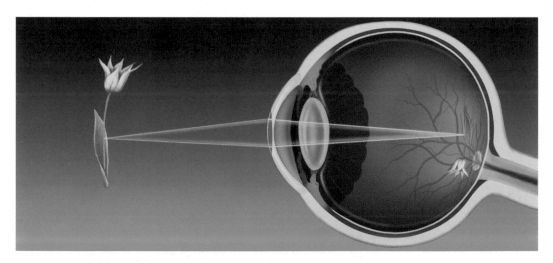

The refraction is corrected for the myopic patient. The subtle change of the
reshaped cornea is shown in purple at the front of the eyeball.

6

After LASIK

Within hours of your surgery, constantly regenerating cells will already be growing over the edge of the corneal flap, helping to "glue" it down. This process takes a few days. Over the next several months, the internal healing process totally seals the flap.

In the interim, however, it's important that you do all you can to make the surgery a success. The moment you leave the LASIK center, you are encouraged to take an active role in your body's healing process by following a specific regimen prescribed by your ophthalmologist.

Your Self-Care Regimen

Follow these recommended guidelines to promote safe and rapid healing.

- Rest. It is a well-documented fact that more healing takes place when patients are sleeping than when they are awake.

- Keep your eyes well lubricated for rapid recovery and enhanced comfort. Particularly in dry climates or air-conditioned environments, apply nonpreserved lubricant eyedrops frequently. Some patients may need these drops every half hour for the first few days, and every couple of hours for a few weeks after that. Your surgeon can recommend a good brand.

- Wear high-quality sunglasses with ultraviolet protection. It is normal to experience increased sensitivity to light at first. This condition will improve.

- Avoid rubbing your eyes for a few days. The corneal flap needs time to adhere evenly without being disturbed.

- Avoid rough contact sports for the first week, for the same reason.

- Avoid swimming, surfing, and hot tubs for at least one week to prevent contact with unwanted germs and bacteria that could cause infection before the corneal flap has totally healed.

- Showers and baths are fine, but avoid getting water and shampoo directly in your eyes for the first few days.

- Avoid dusty or smoky environments for several days.

- Avoid eye makeup for one week.

- It is a good idea to not plan on driving until your vision has improved. It may be the next day or it may take a few days before you feel comfortable enough to drive.

I think LASIK is the tip of the iceberg. I believe eyeglasses will be totally obsolete in twenty years. Our grandchildren will look at eyeglasses the way we look at monocles and whalebone girdles.

Dr. Robert Maloney

Postoperative Appointment Schedule

Keeping your follow-up appointments is as important as sticking to your self-care regimen. Your doctor needs to follow the

Purpose of Appointment	Time Frame Following LASIK Procedure
To ensure that there is no evidence of infection, that the flap is healing properly, and to remove the bandage contact lens (if one was used)	1 day
To ensure that your eye is healing properly	1 week to 1 month
To measure your visual progress and to consider enhancement treatment (if necessary)	3 to 6 months
To measure the stability of your result, check your eye pressure, and assess your general eye health	12 months, at your annual exam

progress of your healing and may recommend changing your eyedrop regimen. Also, he or she may need to monitor your eye pressure if you are on postoperative anti-inflammatory drops for any length of time; these drops may increase pressure inside the eye, creating a risk for glaucoma.

The LASIK Recovery Cycle

Most patients are genuinely surprised by how quickly their vision improves after LASIK. Although the corneal flap adheres quickly, your eyesight will continue to improve until it finally reaches a point at which it becomes stable. The time it takes to establish visual stability after LASIK varies for each patient. For some, stability can be achieved in a few weeks. For others, stability may take three to six months.

During the first month after surgery, you will probably notice a gradual improvement in your vision. It is common to experience fluctuations in your vision during the first two to three weeks, especially for those with higher corrections.

Patients who have hyperopic LASIK (farsightedness treatment) may notice that their near vision is better than their distance vision at first. This is quite common, and the distance vision will continue to improve during the first month.

For the first three months, it is normal for patients to experience an occasional feeling of "grittiness" in the eye. This is related to dryness on the surface of the eye. The frequent use of lubricant drops will help significantly. People with drier eyes and those who use a computer, read for long hours, drive long distances, or live in low-humidity climates may even notice some minor discomfort and blurring of their vision, particularly toward the end of the day. Also caused by dryness, these conditions will improve over time.

Although many patients notice halos around lights or ghosting of images at night, these symptoms tend to lessen substantially within six months.

Before your vision stabilizes, you may feel more comfortable with a thin pair of eyeglasses—those with low prescription lenses—to assist you with critical distance vision activities, such as driving at night. Patients over forty years of age may require a thin pair of glasses for reading.

7

LASIK Statistics: Your Chances for Success

What are my chances of achieving 20/20 vision with LASIK? This is what every patient wants to know. A better question might be: What is the likelihood that my procedure will be successful, given my refractive error? Although it would be unreasonable to be guaranteed 20/20 eyesight after LASIK surgery, it is absolutely justifiable for you to ask your doctor to predict your chances for a successful outcome.

If you have chosen an experienced surgeon—someone who has performed 1,000 LASIK procedures at the absolute minimum—he or she has most likely performed surgery on a number of patients with vision like yours. Accordingly, you will be able to get an idea of what you can reasonably expect after LASIK.

The Importance of Statistics

Fortunately, now that the LASIK procedure has been around for several years, predicting outcomes can be based on scientific data. If you have found a surgeon who tracks outcomes and compiles statistics (should be based on 1,000 or more LASIK procedures, to be accurate), so much the better. This surgeon's numbers will accurately reflect his or her own experience. Statistics and percentages are useful to patients who want to know what kind of vision they can realistically expect after surgery. But these statistics can also be confusing and misleading. For example, when a surgeon talks about the percentage of LASIK patients who achieved 20/20 vision, this might include all patients. Or, it might be limited to those patients who had *only* the initial LASIK procedure (no enhancements). Meanwhile, other surgeons prefer to use 20/40 as the baseline. Since patients will find inconsistencies from center to center on how this information is presented, it is crucial to pay attention to what the numbers are really telling you.

The Statistics to Know

As a patient, what are the important statistics for you to know, and how can you interpret outcomes? First of all, you likely want to know your chances of achieving at least 20/40 vision. This is a key number since 20/40 vision is required to drive legally without eyeglasses or contacts. Second, you probably also want to know your chances of achieving optimal 20/20 vision. Third, you may wish to know the likelihood of needing an enhancement procedure after the initial surgery.

All of the above numbers will vary according to the surgeon you choose and your prescription. For example, patients with higher degrees of nearsightedness or farsightedness are more likely to need an enhancement procedure.

Statistical Outcomes According to Refraction

To accurately predict LASIK outcomes, Dr. Ernest W. Kornmehl conducted a study of 1,630 eyes. His research findings for each procedure follow. Listed according to refractive error, these statistics give an indication of the results to expect from an experienced surgeon.

Keep in mind that the patients in these statistics who do not achieve 20/20 vision without correction are usually still pleased with their results. They can do most things without eyeglasses or contacts, including drive a car. And when it is absolutely necessary for them to fine-tune their vision, they can wear eyeglasses.

Myopia

Mild Myopia

A patient with mild myopia, or nearsightedness, has a nearly 100 percent chance of achieving 20/40 vision or better and being able to drive without eyeglasses or contacts. The chance of achieving 20/20 vision without correction is 98 percent, but this statistic includes patients who require an enhancement procedure, as well as those who do not. The chance that a patient with mild myopia will need an enhancement procedure is 1 percent. Mild myopia is defined as less than −3.00 diopters, with or without astigmatism.

Moderate Myopia

After the initial procedure, nearly 100 percent of patients with moderate myopia achieve 20/40 vision or better. Of these, 88 percent achieve 20/20 vision or better. There is a 3 percent chance of needing an enhancement procedure if you fall into this category. After undergoing an enhancement, almost 100 percent of patients see 20/40 or better and 96 percent see 20/20 or better. Moderate myopia is defined as a refractive error between –3.00 and –6.00 diopters.

Severe Myopia

These patients have a 99 percent chance of seeing 20/40 or better after the initial procedure. Patients with severe myopia have a 6 to 8 percent chance of needing an enhancement procedure, after which they have a 99 percent chance of seeing 20/40 or better and a 90 percent chance of seeing 20/20 or better. Severe myopia is defined as a refractive error between –6.00 and –9.00 diopters.

A common misconception among patients in their late 40s and mid-50s is that they'll have perfect vision—far and near—after LASIK. They will need glasses for small print, unless they receive monovision—one eye corrected for distance and one for close up vision.

Dr. Ernest Kornmehl

Extreme Myopia

Patients with extreme myopia have an 89 percent chance of achieving 20/40 vision or better after the initial procedure. Because of the high level of correction, approximately 12 to 16 percent of this group will need enhancements. After enhancement, 77 percent of patients will have 20/20 vision or better.

Many patients with extreme myopia do well. However, other variables such as the thickness and the steepness of the cornea come into play. Patients in this group need to thoroughly discuss the risks and benefits of LASIK, as well as other options, with their doctor. Although enhancement rates are higher in this group of patients, there may be limitations on what can be done due to other variables in the eye. Extreme myopia is considered a refractive error higher than –9.00 diopters.

Astigmatism

Patients with mild astigmatism can expect nearly identical outcomes and enhancement percentages to those patients with myopia only. The presence of moderate or high degrees of preoperative astigmatism will reduce your chance of achieving 20/20 vision after the initial procedure, making it more likely that you will want to have an enhancement. Mild astigmatism is defined as a refractive error of 1.00 diopter or less.

Hyperopia

The statistics on LASIK outcomes for patients with hyperopia come from a multicenter trial that was conducted for FDA approval of an excimer laser called the VISX Star S2. The participating LASIK surgeons treated patients with hyperopia in the range of +1.00 to +6.00 diopters. In this study, after the initial LASIK procedure 91 percent of the patients achieved 20/40 vision or better, and 53 percent saw 20/20 without eyeglasses.

Patients treated for hyperopia should be aware that their healing time is slightly longer than for patients with myopia, and the chance that they will need an enhancement is slightly higher. These numbers are variable, depending on the patient's original prescription and the skill and experience level of the surgeon.

8

Risks and Complications

Just as all surgical procedures carry risks, so does a LASIK procedure. The good news is, when LASIK is done by an experienced surgeon, the risk of complications is quite low. In fact, LASIK is considered one of the safest surgeries performed today when performed by a reputable surgeon.

Still, it's important to understand the risks and possible complications. Once you understand them, you will be able to determine for yourself whether the potential benefits of LASIK outweigh the risks.

Improper Screening

Most LASIK complications are preventable. The most common reason for complications following LASIK surgery is improper screening of the surgery candidate. For example, an inexperienced surgeon may recommend surgery for a patient who has abnormally large pupils. However, an experienced ophthalmologist may advise such a patient against having LASIK during a careful, preoperative examination. As discussed earlier, there are many reasons to turn down a patient. That is why it's important to choose a surgeon based on his or her experience—not on the cheapest fee available.

Possible Complications

Undercorrection

Undercorrection results when the desired change in your refractive error, or focusing ability, is not fully achieved after the LASIK procedure. A slight undercorrection will not seriously affect your vision and may even be desirable in nearsighted patients over forty to help with their reading vision. More significant undercorrections may require an enhancement procedure, which is usually included in the original LASIK cost if performed within the first year.

Undercorrection happens more often in patients with higher levels of nearsightedness, farsightedness, or astigmatism. This makes sense if you think in terms of how much sculpting, or reshaping, the laser has to do. For example, a patient with less than −2.00 diopters of myopia has about a 1 percent chance of needing an enhancement procedure because of an under-correction. On the other hand, a patient with more than −9.00 diopters of myopia has about a 10 percent chance of requiring an enhancement procedure due to undercorrection.

Surgeons who use consistent techniques and constantly analyze their outcomes have significantly lower incidences of undercorrection. This is another reason why it is important to find a surgeon who tracks LASIK outcomes, as discussed earlier. If your doctor keeps an up-to-date database of at least 1,000 proce-dures, he or she will be able to show you the likelihood of needing retreatment, based on your own degree and type of refractive error.

Overcorrection

Less common than undercorrection, *overcorrection* results when the refractive error is changed more than was intended. An initial, or temporary, overcorrection may occur and usually rights itself in the first month. Following a treatment for farsightedness, an overcorrection would make you temporarily nearsighted. In this case, your distance vision would be somewhat blurred and your near vision rather good. Following a nearsighted treatment, an overcorrection would make it more difficult for you to see objects up close. Patients can manage these temporary overcorrections by wearing glasses until they resolve.

There are fewer permanent over- corrections than permanent undercorrections. A significant overcorrection can be treated with an enhancement procedure as well. Overcorrection enhancements are usually performed three to six months following the initial treatment, after your vision has stabilized.

Induced Astigmatism

In rare circumstances, significant astigmatism results after the initial LASIK surgery. *Induced astigmatism* causes blurred vision. It can be treated with either an overcorrection or an undercorrection enhancement, if necessary. Most people can tolerate small degrees of astigmatism. However, if your vision is blurred because of a refractive error after LASIK and does not meet your expectations, there is a 99 percent chance that it can be corrected with enhancement.

Dry Eye

As detailed earlier, it is not uncommon for patients to experience a feeling of "grittiness" in the eye following LASIK.

This is a common side effect from the surgery that will usually disappear over the first three to six months. The use of nonpreserved lubricating eyedrops, or artificial tears, will help to speed healing and alleviate the symptoms of dry eye.

However, persistent dry eye is also a potential complication of LASIK. This is especially true if you experienced dry eye before LASIK, either with contact lenses or eyeglasses, or if you are taking birth control pills or going through menopause. For dry eye that persists, your doctor may recommend blocking your tear drainage canals with tiny silicone punctum plugs. This brief, painless procedure prevents your natural tears from draining away too quickly and results in better lubrication of the eye.

Patients need to understand LASIK's potential risks as well as the benefits. Prior to performing the procedure, I need to know that the patient truly wants the surgery, rather than having a spouse or significant other pushing them into it.

Dr. Ernest Kornmehl

Corneal Abrasion

Approximately 1 to 5 percent of LASIK patients develop a small *corneal abrasion,* or scrape, caused by friction of the microkeratome. The incidence of corneal abrasion depends on the type of microkeratome used. Despite excellent surgical technique and well-lubricated eyes during the flap-making process, a small breakdown in the epithelium, the thin outer layer of the cornea, may occur as the microkeratome makes the corneal flap.

If this happens, your surgeon will place a very thin bandage contact lens on the eye. The bandage lens improves comfort, promotes healing, and can be removed in one to five days. The abrasions always heal, usually in one to three days. But, it may take up to ten days to achieve your best vision if the abrasion is located centrally.

While the abrasion is healing, your vision will be blurred—as if you are looking through a scratched pair of eyeglasses. If the corneal abrasion is significant, the surgeon may decide to postpone doing LASIK on the other eye for one or two weeks so the first eye will have a chance to heal and your vision will be able to clear up. Chances are likely, if you got a corneal abrasion in one eye, the same thing will happen in your other eye when it undergoes LASIK.

Night Glare, Halos, and Starbursts

Many patients who wear eyeglasses or contacts have experienced these symptoms at night or in dim light conditions. When the pupil dilates, peripheral light rays (rays coming in from the sides) scatter more before they reach the retina. This scattering results in glare, halos, and starbursts. It is important to tell your surgeon about these problems *prior* to your LASIK surgery.

Some patients experience these same symptoms following LASIK surgery, especially if the pupil dilates beyond the treatment zone. Although these symptoms do not necessarily interfere with visual sharpness as measured on the Snellen eye chart, they can be bothersome in dim light conditions such as driving at night.

While some patients may see halos or a ghosting of images at night during the first month following treatment, it is quite uncommon for these side effects to interfere with their activities. The effects usually improve in the first three months, and the overwhelming majority of significant glare problems disappear on their own by six months.

There are treatment options for patients who experience persistent glare, halos, or starbursts. Weak prescription night glasses can help, as can the use of eyedrops at dusk that reduce the size of the pupils.

The probability of having these symptoms after LASIK is difficult to predict. Some patients with large pupils, more severe refractive errors, and astigmatism may be somewhat more prone to glare and halo effects. Special programs for the laser that allow for larger treatment zones can help reduce the chance of these problems. The newest microkeratomes that allow for larger corneal flap sizes may also help to reduce one type of glare.

Loss of Best Corrected Vision

A small number of patients experience a slight loss of visual acuity following LASIK surgery. Loss of best corrected vision means that, even with eyeglasses, you lose some of the visual crispness and clarity you had when you wore eyeglasses or contacts prior to LASIK. You may no longer be able to read the 20/20 line on the Snellen eye chart. Loss of best corrected vision can be due to irregular healing or an irregular flap and may improve over the first year. Careful surgical technique and good follow-up care will help minimize the incidence of this problem.

In extremely rare cases, a reduction in best corrected vision occurs when patients develop diffuse *lamellar keratitis* (an uncommon inflammatory reaction that occurs between the corneal flap and the underlying stroma) or persistent *striae* (wrinkles or folds in the flap). Less than 1 percent of patients will experience a reduction of vision as a result. Most of the time these conditions can be reversed with surgery.

Central Island

Another potential complication from LASIK that reduces vision is a *central island*. A central island is a small raised area in your cornea's treatment zone. Central islands often disappear spontaneously after several months, but some require an enhancement procedure in which the corneal flap is lifted and a small amount of excimer laser energy is delivered to the raised area. When the central island is removed by additional laser treatment, crisp vision usually returns.

Your surgeon will diagnose a central island by using a corneal topographer, the device that produces a digitized contour map of the corneal surface.

Some excimer lasers have special software that distributes additional pulses centrally, along with the regular treatment for the refractive error, to help prevent central islands.

Corneal Flap Complications

For experienced surgeons, corneal flap complications are rare. If they occur, they tend to occur at the time of surgery.

This complication is characterized by a flap that is too small, too thin, or irregularly shaped. If there are problems with the flap, your surgeon may elect not to go ahead with LASIK but to perform it instead at a later date, after the eye heals. Allowing the cornea to heal for three to four months is usually adequate. Typically, you might experience glare, shadowing, or blurred vision while the flap is healing.

The corneal flap could also be created without a hinge, although this is not likely with today's newer microkeratomes. Sometimes, postoperatively, the corneal flap may shift slightly.

This is why it is important, especially during the first few hours, not to rub your eyes and to keep them well lubricated.

If the flap shifts slightly, wrinkles could form. If these striae are present in the center of the cornea, they may distort vision and require smoothing out. This is done by lifting the flap and "ironing" them out with a special instrument. When treated early, striae can usually be completely removed. Occasionally, however, they can be difficult to treat, and rarely they can lead to a reduction in best corrected vision.

While any problem with the corneal flap can result in the loss of best corrected vision, the good news is that the overwhelming majority of flap-related complications can be easily managed. They rarely have serious long-term consequences. However, it may take several months for your best vision to be restored following correction of the problem. If a flap complication were to occur, a truly experienced surgeon would be able to manage it appropriately.

Among experienced LASIK surgeons, the incidence of flap-related complications that affect vision significantly is less than 0.5 percent.

Epithelial Ingrowth

Another rare complication, *epithelial ingrowth,* is produced when the surface cells of the cornea grow underneath the corneal flap during the first month following LASIK surgery. These cells occasionally cause blurred vision or irritation. Epithelial ingrowth is easy to identify and is treated by gently lifting the flap and clearing away the trapped epithelial cells.

Regression

Regression refers to the tendency of the eye to drift back slightly toward the original refractive error. This occurs more commonly in LASIK patients with higher amounts of myopia, hyperopia, or astigmatism.

If significant regression occurs, you may require either low prescription eyeglasses for night driving or an enhancement procedure to "tune up" the original treatment, provided your cornea is thick enough to allow retreatment. Enhancements for regression are usually performed three to six months after the original procedure to allow time for the patient's vision to stabilize.

Diffuse Lamellar Keratitis

Diffuse lamellar keratitis (DLK)—also known as "Sands of the Sahara" syndrome—is a noninfectious inflammation that sometimes occurs between the corneal flap and the underlying stroma. Extremely rare, DLK leaves small white deposits underneath the corneal flap after LASIK. The doctor typically observes this condition the day after surgery using a slit lamp microscope. You may have no symptoms, or you may notice some haziness in your vision.

The chances of DLK can be significantly reduced by your surgeon maintaining meticulously clean conditions between the flap and the underlying stroma during the LASIK procedure. Also, following LASIK you will receive a *topical corticosteroid,* a medicated eye drop used to suppress inflammation. You will be instructed to apply these drops at least four days following the procedure, since DLK peaks two to five days after surgery. Most cases of DLK respond to treatment with corticosteroid drops. More severe cases may require that the surgeon lift the corneal flap and irrigate beneath it to remove the inflammatory cells. When recognized early and treated properly, DLK rarely affects vision in the long run. In severe cases, DLK will cause a loss of best corrected vision.

Infection

Although infection is the most feared complication, it is extremely rare. As with any surgery, proper technique is the best way to avoid infection. If your eye does get infected, it will likely occur during the first forty-eight to seventy-two hours after LASIK. This is why it is so important to avoid any contact with substances that may cause infection, such as eye makeup, hot tubs, and swimming pools for the first week. It is also essential to go to all of your follow-up visits, even if everything seems fine. To prevent infection, you will use antibiotic drops postoperatively. Starting these drops two days before surgery can further reduce your risk.

Conclusion

LASIK vision correction is the most popular refractive surgery performed today. Its reputation is well deserved, as people discover that LASIK delivers good vision safely when it is performed by experienced, skilled surgeons. Perhaps more telling than the general public's enthusiasm for LASIK, however, is the widespread acceptance the procedure has gained among professionals in the fields of ophthalmology and optometry.

What does the future hold for people who could benefit from laser vision correction? Currently in the United States, myopia, hyperopia, and astigmatism have all been approved for treatment, but only for refractive errors that fall within certain parameters. Newer laser technology is being developed that expands these parameters, which will make it possible to treat patients with more severe vision problems in the future.

The issue of gradually losing one's near vision after age forty, or presbyopia, is still looming. A number of medical research efforts are now underway to develop procedures that could restore near vision in the vast majority of aging patients. Some of the research involves new techniques to reshape the cornea, others to restore the function of the focusing muscles of the eye, and still others that concentrate on the lens itself.

Newer lasers entering the marketplace now offer customizable programs that allow surgeons to treat patients with irregular corneas on a patient-by-patient basis.

Finally, there are new tracking devices that lock the excimer laser beam onto the patient's eye. If the patient's eye moves, the laser moves with it. This innovation should benefit patients who find it difficult to fix their eyes in one place and those who require particularly long treatments.

In its current state, LASIK has proven to be a life-changing experience for many. However, the decision to have LASIK is an important one that ultimately only you can make. We hope to have given you information that will help you make sound decisions based on facts, not on hopes or misconceptions.

Appendix

Other Refractive Procedures

If it turns out that you are not a good candidate for LASIK, you and your doctor may wish to consider other surgical options. One of the procedures listed below may be appropriate.

Photorefractive Keratectomy (PRK)

Laser vision correction with PRK is very similar to LASIK. The biggest difference is that no microkeratome is used and no corneal flap is created. Instead, the excimer laser makes its correction directly on the surface of your cornea, removing the central epithelium and *Bowman's layer* (the second corneal layer) in the process. This results in several days of potential discomfort and blurred vision until the epithelium regenerates.

The actual laser part of the procedure takes twenty to ninety seconds. At the end of the procedure, a clear-bandage contact lens is placed over your eye to help keep you comfortable while the corneal epithelium regenerates (usually three to five days).

A typical PRK procedure takes about three to five minutes per eye. Operating on just one eye, or both eyes on the same day, is a decision to be made by the patient after discussing the pros and cons with the surgeon. Because the return of functional vision is prolonged under PRK, most surgeons prefer to wait at least one week before operating on the second eye.

Patients with certain corneal problems, such as an irregular corneal surface or a thin cornea, may be better candidates for PRK than for LASIK. The ultimate visual results are similar with PRK, although the recovery is somewhat prolonged in comparison.

One advantage of PRK over LASIK is that there is no risk of flap complications since no corneal flap is created. However, other potential complications of PRK are similar to those of LASIK. They include undercorrection, overcorrection, induced astigmatism, dry eye, haze, night glare and halos, loss of best corrected vision, infection or severe inflammation, and regression. Other disadvantages of PRK include the need for anti-inflammatory eyedrops for three months and the risk of corneal haze or scarring.

Regression occurs when a patient appears to be adequately treated on the first few postoperative visits, but over the next several weeks to months begins to return toward the original prescription. The amount of regression is usually small; however, occasionally it is visually significant and requires an enhancement procedure. The enhancement procedure is usually performed six to nine months after the original procedure. The time period before the return of optimal vision is significantly longer than with an enhancement after LASIK.

Intacs Corneal Ring Segments

Approved by the FDA in April 1999, *Intacs corneal ring segments* offer patients with mild myopia and minimal astigmatism another option for correcting their nearsightedness. Currently, the rings are approved for correction of nearsightedness up to 3.00

diopters in patients twenty-one years or older who have no more than 1.00 diopter of astigmatism. Note: this procedure does *not* correct astigmatism. Patients who have astigmatism—even less than 1.00 diopter—need to understand they will be astigmatic postoperatively. Intacs are newer than LASIK and PRK, so they don't yet have a track record like the other two procedures.

With Intacs, two small plastic ring segments are inserted in the peripheral cornea through small incisional channels. A temporary suture is then used to close the incision. The rings cause the central cornea to flatten. The rings are intended to be permanent, but they may be removed if the patient wishes to reverse the correction.

In clinical trials, when the rings were removed, many patients' eyes went back to their preoperative state. In some patients, they did not. Because some patients' eyes did not return exactly to their preoperative condition, the FDA will not allow the use of the term *reversible*, but Intacs are certainly *removable* if desired.

Intacs insertion takes slightly longer than LASIK, roughly fifteen minutes per eye under anesthetic drops. The recovery of clear vision takes slightly longer than LASIK. In addition, patients tend to experience more postoperative discomfort.

The cost of Intacs is roughly equal to, or more than, LASIK in most centers. Removal of the rings, either for fine-tuning the result or from dissatisfaction, is accomplished with a second surgery. The segments are removed, the eyes are allowed to heal, and an alternate procedure (such as LASIK, PRK, or a change in ring size) may be performed once the eyes have healed. The treatment range for Intacs is currently very limited.

Radial Keratotomy (RK)

Until excimer lasers became available, *radial keratotomy (RK)* was the most commonly performed refractive procedure for nearsighted patients. With the aid of a high-powered microscope, the surgeon makes a series of radial microscopic incisions (usually between four and eight) on the surface of the cornea to reduce its curvature. This procedure was well suited for patients with low myopia and has been used for over twenty-five years. One form of RK, *mini-RK*, is still used occasionally for very minute degrees of nearsightedness, such as those resulting from slight undercorrections in LASIK or following cataract or clear lens extraction surgery.

Although outdated by excimer laser techniques, RK is still an effective procedure. It is used in those areas of the world that do not have access to the much more expensive laser technologies.

Astigmatic Keratotomy (AK)

Astigmatic keratotomy (AK) is similar to RK, but its purpose is to correct only astigmatism. Usually, one or two incisions are made in the peripheral cornea to make it more round (as if loosening the laces on a football). This procedure is often combined with RK and has a similar long track record.

AK is a reasonable procedure for correcting pure astigmatism (patients without coexisting nearsightedness or farsightedness) with results that are almost as good as those with LASIK and PRK. AK can also be used to enhance the results of LASIK and PRK by correcting small residual amounts of astigmatism. The most frequent use of AK today is to correct astigmatism at the time of lens implant surgery (either cataract or clear lens extraction surgery).

Cataract Surgery

For patients with significant cataracts who are looking to correct their nearsightedness or farsightedness, *cataract surgery* presents the best option. After removing the cataract with ultrasonic power, the surgeon can implant a lens that will reduce or eliminate nearsightedness and farsightedness. With the new toric intraocular lens implants, or in combination with AK, astigmatism can also be treated.

This procedure is not performed on younger patients *without* cataracts because the surgery involves entering the eye and, therefore, slightly increases the risk of more serious complications. The surgery also involves removing the natural crystalline lens, which in young people allows them to focus up close. LASIK, which leaves the lens intact, is a better option for younger patients.

Modern cataract surgery, when performed by an experienced surgeon, can allow patients a recovery period rather similar to that of LASIK. In its most sophisticated form, cataract surgery can be performed with eyedrop anesthesia (just like LASIK or PRK) and require no sutures. An outpatient procedure in skilled hands, it takes twenty minutes or less to complete.

Automated Lamellar Keratoplasty (ALK)

Automated lamellar keratoplasty (ALK) was done on high myopes prior to the invention of the excimer laser. ALK is not performed today. LASIK has essentially replaced ALK because of the increased accuracy and safety afforded by the excimer laser in making the second "cut." ALK is similar to LASIK in that it uses a microkeratome to separate the surface layer of the cornea. This flap is temporarily folded back (similar to the first part of the LASIK procedure), and a thin disc of corneal tissue is removed with a second pass of the microkeratome. ALK, much less precise than LASIK, was associated with a much higher complication rate. It was primarily used to correct large amounts of myopia.

Satisfactory results are not always obtained the first time, and a high percentage of eyes need additional procedures to achieve the desired result. Sometimes an irregular corneal surface results from the procedure, causing some distortion of vision.

Phakic Intraocular Lens (PIOL) Implants

A *phakic intraocular lens (PIOL) implant* may correct either extreme nearsightedness or extreme farsightedness. Unlike cataract surgery, your natural lens is not removed; rather, the implant sits in front of the natural lens. In effect, the PIOL becomes an internal contact lens.

Implantable contact lens technology has arisen out of the incredible advances in modern cataract surgery. Current technology allows ophthalmologists to insert flexible intraocular lenses (used to replace the natural lens after cataract surgery) through extremely small incisions. Some PIOL implants, too, are flexible enough to allow folding as they are inserted through small incision openings.

Because of the slightly increased risk of more serious complications, PIOL implants are reserved for high amounts of nearsightedness or farsightedness—beyond the safe limits of LASIK. In places where this technology is available, surgeons are implanting PIOLs in patients with myopia greater than 12.00 to 15.00 diopters and hyperopia greater than 4.00 to 6.00 diopters. In addition, PIOL implants may be preferable to LASIK in patients who fall within the safe LASIK parameters with regard to their prescription but who have thinner corneas, making the tissue removal aspect of LASIK less desirable.

Despite the excellent outcomes in most cases, complications associated with PIOL implants are currently the biggest concern. Specifically, in the early studies, a small percentage of patients developed cataracts shortly after implantation of one brand of the lens. There is also a small risk of *endophthalmitis* (infection within the eye) because the surgical incision actually enters the eye. This rare complication could lead to a complete loss of vision. Endothelial cell loss with some lens designs is also a concern and is being studied rigorously.

Some ophthalmologists in the United States are currently implanting PIOLs as part of an FDA clinical trial. The procedure holds a lot of promise for extremely nearsighted and farsighted individuals. Ophthalmologists are eager to see how PIOL implants fare in current studies using newer lens designs and implantation techniques. These lenses are currently being used in Europe and South America with very high success rates. The results of the U.S. clinical trial will be presented to the FDA with the hope that it will authorize other eye surgeons to use this exciting new technology.

Bioptics

Bioptics is a combination procedure involving a PIOL implant followed by LASIK. It is recommended for the most extreme levels of myopia and hyperopia when neither technique alone will entirely correct the refractive error. This combined technique can be used to correct over 30.00 diopters of myopia—twice the maximum amount that can be safely corrected with LASIK.

Clear Lens Extraction (CLE)

Clear lens extraction (CLE) involves removing the eye's lens, just like in a cataract operation. This is done with a special ultrasound instrument and may be accompanied by eyedrop anesthesia. A flexible synthetic lens implant of the proper power is then placed inside the eye through an extremely small incision to correct the refractive error. The procedure can be completed without sutures. Visual recovery is quite rapid. As with LASIK, most patients are able to return to work the day following their procedure.

CLE is most commonly performed to treat higher levels of farsightedness in patients over age forty. The optical results are superior to LASIK for these higher corrections. CLE may also be used to correct higher levels of nearsightedness and may be fine-tuned with LASIK if a small refractive error remains. Some surgeons have used CLE to treat extremely nearsighted or farsighted patients who are not candidates for LASIK or PRK.

The major drawbacks of CLE are the risk of postoperative retinal detachment (more of a risk with nearsighted than farsighted patients), and the risks of intraocular surgery (including the potential, albeit uncommon, risk of endophthalmitis).

If both eyes are corrected for distance vision, CLE patients will require reading glasses after their procedure. As with LASIK and PRK, however, monovision corrections are possible with CLE to decrease or even eliminate one's need for reading glasses. Or, a new intraocular lens called the *ARRAY* lens can be implanted at the time of lens extraction. The multifocal ARRAY lens allows you to see both near and far after the operation. For the best results, both eyes should be implanted with the lens. Because of its multifocal capacity, some patients experience a loss of contrast at night and also develop halos around lights. If these symptoms become problematic, the ARRAY lens can be removed and replaced with a conventional lens implant.

Laser Thermal Keratoplasty (LTK)

For low amounts of farsightedness, a technique called *laser thermal keratoplasty* (LTK) is a possible method of thermally changing the shape of the cornea. A special holmium laser is used to deliver laser energy to the peripheral cornea to slightly tighten the fibers and thereby steepen its curvature. The technique seems to work only for low amounts of farsightedness.

In January 2000, the Sunrise Hyperion LTK System received FDA approval for the treatment of hyperopia (0.75 to 2.50 diopters). The procedure takes just a few minutes per eye and is performed with the patient seated. The LTK procedure may also be useful for treating occasional overcorrections from LASIK procedures.

There are two disadvantages of LTK. First is the long time needed for vision to stabilize. This process can take months, requiring multiple pairs of glasses in the interim. The second disadvantage is that the effect wears off in a substantial percentage of patients. A patient in whom the effect wears off either faces having the treatment repeated every year or so, or turns to LASIK for a permanent correction.

Conductive Keratoplasty (CK)

In *conductive keratoplasty (CK)*, a special probe introduces an electrical current to the peripheral cornea, shrinking the corneal fibers. Similar to LTK, this acts like tightening a belt, causing the central cornea to steepen. It is effective for small amounts of hyperopia. The procedure takes less than five minutes and is essentially painless. It may be performed in a doctor's office without the need of a laser suite. The major advantage of CK is its relative safety. Because all the work is done on the peripheral cornea, the risk of central corneal scarring (through the visual axis, or line of sight) is minimal. The visual recovery with CK is fairly quick, although generally somewhat slower than with LASIK. CK is considered by many surgeons to be the next advance over LTK because its effect appears to be permanent.

Surgery for Presbyopia

One of the more exciting areas of ophthalmology is the surgical treatment of presbyopia—the stiffening of the natural lens that decreases near vision as we age. Several devices and surgeries have been tried, all of which attempt to enlarge the circumference of the eye and tighten the fibers that control the focus of the lens. These fibers are thought to stretch and become less effective as we age.

Anterior Ciliary Sclerotomy (ACS)

Anterior ciliary sclerotomy (ACS) is a surgical procedure for relieving presbyopia. Several small incisions are made in the sclera (coating of the eye) directly over the muscle that controls the lens. This procedure expands the circumference of the eye. ACS may be combined with the placement of small silicone plugs into the scleral grooves. These plugs may help the effect last longer.

Scleral Expansion Bands (SEBs)

Scleral expansion bands (SEBs) also may relieve presbyopia. A number of thin silicon bands are implanted in the sclera to expand the equator of the eye in order to restore accommodation.

The theory behind both ACS and SEB is that expansion of the eye will allow increased room for the lens to move normally, enabling the eye to see nearby objects again. These procedures are still being investigated in the United States. To date, there is considerable controversy about both the theory and the effectiveness of ACS and SEB. Until scientific studies show more consistent results, monovision and reading glasses or bifocals are still the best options for treating presbyopia.

Resources

International Society of Refractive Surgery (ISRS)
1180 Springs Centre South Boulevard, Suite 116
Altamonte Springs, FL 32714
Phone (407) 786-7446
www.isrs.org

ISRS is an international organization of eye-care professionals committed to providing scientific research, knowledge, and information to all individuals interested in refractive surgery. The site posts technical articles from current and back issues of the *Journal of Refractive Surgery*. Of interest to consumers is the "Locate an ISRS Doctor" search engine, which lists refractive surgeons by city.

American Academy of Ophthalmology (AAO)
P.O. Box 7424
San Francisco, CA 94120-7424
Phone: (415) 561-8500
www.eyenet.org or www.aao.org

One of the leading organizations for ophthalmologists, AAO offers courses, a scientific journal, conferences, and other educational and professional services to eye doctors. The site posts highly technical articles from the archives of the *Journal of Ophthalmology.* Click on "Find an Eye M.D." to find a list of board-certified ophthalmologists who specialize in refractive surgery.

American Society of Cataract and Refractive Surgery (ASCRS)
4000 Legato Road, Suite 850
Fairfax, VA 22033
Phone (703) 591-2220
www.ascrs.org

ASCRS is an international educational and scientific organization whose 8,000 member ophthalmologists specialize in cataract and refractive surgery. ASCRS members are recognized leaders and innovators in ophthalmic surgery worldwide. This site is geared toward physicians, but it also offers helpful consumer eye-care information. The "Find a Surgeon" feature provides a list of ASCRS member eye surgeons by zip code.

LASIK Institute
750 Washington Street, Box 450
Boston, MA 02111
Phone (617) 636-5754
www.lasikinstitute.org

The LASIK Institute is a nonprofit educational organization dedicated to promoting the best possible understanding and practice of LASIK. The site provides comprehensive, consumer-friendly information about LASIK surgery.

National Eye Institute (NEI)
2020 Vision Place
Bethesda, MD 20892-3655

(301) 496-5248

www.nei.nih.gov

The National Eye Institute (NEI) supports more than 80 percent of the vision research conducted in the United States at approximately 250 medical centers, hospitals, universities, and other institutions. In addition, the Institute conducts studies in its own facilities in Bethesda, Maryland to combat the myriad of eye disorders affecting millions of people worldwide. The site lists current NEI-supported clinical trials and how to participate in them. The web site includes an on-line fact sheet for finding eye-care professionals and a fact sheet on how to obtain financial aid for eye care. NEI also offers free publications that can be ordered on-line.

American Board of Medical Specialties (ABMS)

1007 Church Street, Suite 404

Evanston, IL 60201-5913

Phone Verification on surgeons call: (866) ASK-ABMS

Phone: (847) 491-9091

www.abms.org

The American Board of Medical Specialties (ABMS) is the umbrella organization for the twenty-four approved medical specialty boards in the United States. Established in 1933, the ABMS serves to coordinate the activities of its member boards and to provide information to the public, the government, the profession, and its members concerning issues involving specialization and certification in medicine. The mission of the ABMS to maintain and improve the quality of medical care in the United States by assisting the member boards in their efforts to develop and utilize professional and educational standards for the evaluation and certification of physician specialists.

Federation of State Medical Boards
Federation Place
400 Fuller Wiser Road, Suite 300
Euless, Texas 76039-3855
Phone (817) 868-4000
www.fsmb.org

The Federation of State Medical Boards of the United States, Inc., is a national organization comprised of the 69 medical boards of the United States, the District of Columbia, Puerto Rico, Guam and the U.S. Virgin Islands. The mission is to be a leader in improving the quality, safety and integrity of health care in the United States by promoting high standards for physician licensure and practice. FSMB operates the Federation Physician Data Center, a nationally recognized system for collecting, recording and distributing to state medical boards and other appropriate agencies data on disciplinary actions taken against licensees by the boards and other governmental authorities.

Food and Drug Administration
5600 Fishers Lane (HFE-88)
Rockville, MD 20852
www.fda.gov

The FDA, which oversees the safety of food, cosmetics, medicines, medical devices, and radiation-emitting products, also has a consumer-friendly web site. An entire section devoted to LASIK includes educational articles written for the layperson. Also posted are consumer updates, a list of FDA-approved lasers, a directory for consumer and manufacturer calls and complaints, and links to other on-line FDA manuals and publications.

HealthFinder

www.healthfinder.gov

HealthFinder is a service of the U.S. Department of Health and Human Services. Written for the consumer, the web site features articles on timely health topics, the latest government health news, advice and how-to tips for patients, links to on-line journals, and links to medical databases. The site also posts LASIK-related web resources through keyword search.

Glossary

Ablate: To remove, or vaporize, tissue using laser energy.

Ablation zone: The area of tissue removed by the laser. Also called the treatment zone.

Accommodation: The ability of the eye's lens to fine-tune focus by flexing, becoming more convex or more concave, as needed. Accommodation can compensate for minor focusing problems in younger people whose lens and surrounding muscles are still limber and pliable.

Antibiotic drops: Eyedrops containing medicine that prevents infection by killing or inhibiting harmful bacteria.

Anti-inflammatory drops: Eyedrops containing medicine that counteracts inflammation, which is characterized by redness, heat, pain, and swelling.

Artificial tears: Sterile, nonpreserved eyedrops used to lubricate the eyes the same way tears do.

Astigmatism: A refractive error caused by an asymmetrically shaped cornea. Rather than being spherical in shape, the cornea is shaped like a football, causing light to come to several points of focus instead of meeting at a single point of focus. People with astigmatism experience blurred images or double vision.

Automated lamellar keratoplasty (ALK): An older refractive surgery, developed in 1987, in which the surgeon first creates an extremely thin flap in the uppermost layer of the cornea using a device called a microkeratome, then makes a second pass with the microkeratome to remove additional tissue.

Axis: A measurement of astigmatism, the axis (a line) is the symmetrical center of a curved optical surface.

Benchmarking: The process of tracking statistical outcomes for the purpose of predicting future outcomes. With LASIK, statistics from 1,000 or more procedures can provide a good basis for benchmarking.

Best corrected vision: The best possible vision achieved with corrective lenses.

Blended vision: See monovision.

Board-certified: Physicians who have undergone the additional education, internships, residencies, and examinations required for certification.

Cataract: Clouding of the lens within the eye causing decreased vision.

Central island: A treatable complication from LASIK in which a small raised area in the center of the cornea's treatment zone results from having received less laser energy than the surrounding tissue. Central islands can cause distorted vision.

Central lamellar keratitis (CLK): An inflammation on the cornea between the corneal flap and the stroma. This rare complication of LASIK is characterized by small deposits under the corneal flap that can sometimes damage the underlying stroma enough to affect vision and require an enhancement procedure.

Constrict: To become smaller.

Cornea: The outer, dome-shaped, transparent part of the eye that bulges out at the front of the eyeball and covers the iris and pupil. Its curvature causes light to bend. The cornea provides most of the eye's focusing power. It is the only part of the eye on which LASIK is performed.

Corneal topographer: An instrument that creates a three-dimensional map of the cornea using computerized analysis.

Cryolathe: A mechanical lathe used to grind a frozen corneal disc into a new shape before it is replaced on the eye.

Crystalline lens: See lens.

Cylinder: One of three measures in an eyeglass prescription. It indicates whether astigmatism is present, and to what degree.

Diffuse lamellar keratitis (DLK): A potential complication of LASIK, also known as "sands of the Sahara" syndrome. DLK is a noninfectious inflammation that arises between the corneal flap and the underlying stroma.

Dilate: To become larger, as when the pupil enlarges in very dim light conditions.

Diopter: A measurement of refractive error. Hyperopia is measured in terms of positive diopters. Myopia is measured in terms of negative diopters.

Disease neutral: Something that neither prevents diseases nor affects the treatment of diseases. LASIK is considered disease neutral.

Dry eye: A condition characterized by corneal dryness due to inadequate tear production.

Endothelium: The innermost layer of the cornea, a single cell thick, that helps regulate the cornea's hydration.

Enhancement procedure: A secondary treatment with the excimer laser to fine-tune one's visual acuity after the initial LASIK procedure. Enhancements take place after vision has stabilized, usually two to three months after LASIK. Enhancements usually do not require making a new corneal flap.

Epithelial ingrowth: A potential complication of LASIK produced when corneal surface cells, or epithelium, grow underneath the corneal flap during the first month following surgery. The condition is often easily diagnosed and treated.

Epithelium: The thin, protective, outermost surface of the cornea. It is made up of the same kind of cells that cover most of the body. The epithelium grows rapidly and continually regenerates.

Excimer laser: The type of laser used in refractive surgery to remove corneal tissue. It emits highly precise pulses of ultraviolet light to break up tissue, one molecular layer at a time, vaporizing it without generating heat that could damage surrounding tissue.

Eyelid speculum: A device placed between the upper and lower eyelids to keep the patient from blinking.

Ghosting: The appearance of double images or shadows around images. Ghosting is sometimes experienced by people with astigmatism, and can also result from irregular healing of the corneal surface after LASIK.

Glaucoma: A disorder of the eye characterized by an increase of pressure within the eyeball.

Halo: A complication of LASIK in which the patient sees additional rings around lights at night. Halos often decrease with time.

Haze: Scarring of the corneal stroma, or corneal bed. Significant haze is an extremely rare complication of LASIK.

Herpes simplex: A recurrent viral infection of the eye characterized by a painful sore on the eyelid or surface of the eye. It causes inflammation of the cornea and can lead to blindness.

Hyperopia: Also known as farsightedness, hyperopia occurs when the eyeball is too short from front to back, or the eye's focusing mechanism is too weak, causing light rays to be focused behind, rather than on, the retina. People with hyperopia see objects at a distance more clearly than close up, but may have difficulty with both.

Induced astigmatism: A rare complication of LASIK in which astigmatism develops after the initial surgery. Most people can tolerate a small degree of astigmatism. In more serious cases, induced astigmatism can be treated with an enhancement, if necessary.

Inflammation: A localized response to an injury that results in redness, heat, pain, and swelling, and can result in tissue damage if left untreated.

Informed consent: A legal form the patient will be asked to sign after thoroughly discussing the risks, benefits, alternative options, and possible complications of LASIK.

Intraocular pressure: The pressure exerted by the fluid within the eye that gives it its round, firm shape.

Iris: The colored ring of tissue in the eye that is behind the cornea and in front of the lens. The muscles of the iris can adjust the size of the opening, or pupil, to allow for larger or smaller amounts of light to enter the eye.

Keratectomy: Surgical removal of any part of the cornea. In the context of LASIK, keratectomy is the flap-making part of the procedure.

Keratomileusis: Any process of carving, or reshaping, the cornea.

Lamellar: An adjective meaning "layered." Lamellar corneal surgery corrects focusing errors by removing or reshaping some of the corneal layers.

LASIK: An acronym for laser-assisted in situ keratomileusis. In LASIK, a small instrument called a microkeratome creates an extremely thin, hinged flap on the surface of the cornea. After the flap is gently lifted back, the surgeon reshapes the corneal stroma using an excimer laser. The corneal flap is then replaced, and it quickly adheres. LASIK is a safe and pain-free form of refractive eye surgery that has proven to be highly successful and popular.

Latent hyperopia: An age-related phenomenon in which mild farsightedness increases after age thirty or forty.

Lens: The globe-shaped natural lens of the eye, located behind the iris, that helps fine-tune the angle of light to bring it to a point of focus on the retina. As the lens becomes less flexible with age, its ability to refine focus gradually decreases.

Microkeratome: The instrument a surgeon uses to create the corneal flap in the uppermost layer of the cornea during the LASIK procedure.

Monovision: A process by which the surgeon corrects one's dominant eye for seeing at a distance and one's nondominant eye for seeing objects close up.

Myopia: Also known as nearsightedness, myopia is due to a cornea that has too much curvature, or an eyeball that is too long, causing light to be focused in front of, rather than on, the retina. People with myopia have difficulty seeing objects at a distance.

Nomogram: The surgeon's formula entered into the laser's computer calculation to further refine the manufacturer's recommended settings.

Nonfreeze keratomileusis: A process of reshaping the corneal disc directly on the eye without having to remove the disc and freeze it for the purpose of reshaping, as was done in early lamellar surgeries, precursors to LASIK.

Ophthalmology: The field of science dealing with diseases and conditions of the eye.

Ophthalmologist: A medical doctor specializing in the diagnosis and medical or surgical treatment of eye diseases.

Optic nerve: A bundle of nerve fibers, about the diameter of a pencil, that connects to the nerve fiber layer of the retina and terminates in the brain. The optic nerve carries the visual messages from the photoreceptors of the retina to the brain, where images are created and processed.

Optometrist: An eye-care professional specializing in the examination, diagnosis, treatment, management, and prevention of diseases and disorders of the eye.

Orthokeratology: A technique for treating myopia using a series of rigid contact lenses to reshape the cornea. The lenses apply pressure to the sides of the cornea, flattening them.

Overcorrection: A complication of LASIK, overcorrection results when the amount of correction resulting from the LASIK procedure is more than intended.

Peripheral vision: The ability to see objects and movement outside of, or on the periphery of, one's direct line of vision.

Photoablation: The process of removing, or vaporizing, tissue by means of laser energy.

Photorefractive keratectomy (PRK): A type of laser vision correction that reshapes the cornea by ablating, or vaporizing, the corneal tissue one microscopic layer at a time using an excimer laser. Unlike LASIK, in which a hinged corneal flap is first made and lifted back, exposing the corneal bed, the sculpting process used in PRK removes the outer (epithelial) layer of the cornea as the laser energy works its way down to the corneal bed.

Presbyopia: Often confused with farsightedness, presbyopia (literally, "old eyes") is the age-dependent need for reading glasses or bifocals, caused by the decreasing ability of the eye's lens and surrounding muscles to fine-tune focus.

Punctum plugs: Used in the treatment of dry eye, these tiny silicone plugs are inserted into the tear-drainage openings of one's eyelid to delay the drainage of natural tears so the eyes will stay moist.

Pupil: The small black dot, or opening, in the center of the iris. The pupil changes its diameter in response to changes in lighting.

Radial keratotomy (RK): A form of refractive surgery in which the surgeon alters the shape of the cornea by making thin incisions around the cornea in a spoke-like pattern. The incisions cause the central portion of the cornea to flatten, treating myopia and astigmatism.

Refract: To bend, as when light passes through a curved shape such as a cornea or lens.

Refractive error: The degree to which one's eye is able to refract, or bend, light. People with refractive errors (focusing problems) are nearsighted or farsighted, and may have astigmatism as well.

Refractive surgery: Any type of surgery that changes the focusing power of the eye in order to correct a refractive error. LASIK is a type of refractive surgery that corrects the eye's focusing ability by reshaping the curvature of the cornea.

Regression: A potential complication of LASIK in which the eye tends to drift back, or regress, toward its original refractive error.

Retina: The light-sensitive layer of cells on the inner back surface of the eye that processes light and functions much like film in a camera. The retina converts light into electrical impulses that are transmitted along the optic nerve to the brain, which interprets the impulses as images.

Sclera: The tough "white" of the eye that makes up five-sixths of the outer layer of the eyeball. Along with the cornea, it protects the eyeball.

Snellen eye chart: The standard eye chart used by optometrists and ophthalmologists to determine visual acuity.

Sphere: One of three measurements taken during an eye examination to arrive at one's eyeglass prescription. The sphere measures where the eye focuses light—on the retina (normal vision) in front of the retina (myopia), or behind the retina (hyperopia).

Starburst: A visual aberration in which the patient sees rays radiating from lights viewed at night. Starbursts may be seen by people who wear eyeglasses and contact lenses, and are sometimes experienced by patients who have undergone LASIK.

Striae: Wrinkles or folds in the corneal flap that are a potential complication of LASIK. Striae can be smoothed out and corrected if treated early.

Stroma: The strong, fibrous layer that makes up 90 percent of the cornea's thickness and provides the cornea with its structure and shape. Also called the stromal bed, this is the part of the cornea sculpted with the laser in LASIK surgery.

Tonometry: A procedure for measuring intraocular pressure, or the pressure inside the eye.

Topical corticosteroid: A medicated eye drop that prevents inflammation of the eye tissue following LASIK surgery.

Undercorrection: A complication of LASIK, undercorrection results when the amount of correction resulting from the LASIK procedure is less than intended. Most undercorrections can be treated with an enhancement procedure.

Visual acuity: The sharpness or clarity of vision that enables one to distinguish fine details and shapes.

Vitreous humor: The gel-like substance, composed of about 99 percent water, that fills the main cavity of the eye between the lens and the retinal wall.

Index

blurring
  caused by epithelial
  ingrowth, 71
  post-LASIK, 53, 68
  of vision, 8, 40, 42
board certification, 29
Bowman's layer, 17, 76

C

cataract surgery, 80
cataracts, 24, 40
central island, 70
CK (conductive keratoplasty),
  84, 85
CLE (clear lens extraction), 83,
  84
clear lens extraction (CLE), 83,
  84
clinical trials, 17, 32, 33, 47
  intacs corneal ring segments,
  77
cold sores, 40
collagen vascular disease, 24
common vision problems, 7–9
  see also **refractive error**
complication rates, 32
complications, 24, 44, 64–73
conductive keratoplasty (CK),
  84, 85
consultation, 38-48
  with former patients, 31
  initial, 38, 39
  with surgeon, 38, 49
contact lenses, 12, 13, 67
  after LASIK, 46
  as bandage, 67

instructions prior to LASIK,
38, 39
rigid, 13
rigid gas permeable, 39
toric, 39
cornea, 4, 6
  abnormally structured, 24, 41
  curvature, 4, 7
  flattening, 8
  fluid content regulation, 4
  infection, 13
  inflammation, 40
  layers of, 4, 17
  measurement, 41
  oval shaped, 8
  reference marks, 51
  reshaping to correct vision,
  14–20
  scarring, 13, 46, 85
  sculpting, 18, 20
  stabilization, 39
  thickness, 22, 24, 41
  warped, 13, 22
corneal
  abrasion, 67, 68
  dystrophies, 24
  flap, 52, 56, 57, 67
  haze, 16, 77
  scarring, 13, 46, 85
  topographer, 41, 70
  transplant, 46
  trauma prevention, 54
corneal flap
  complications, 70, 71
  shifting, 70
cylinder measurement, 11

Index

intraocular, 83
light
  control, 4, 5
  refraction, 7
  sensitivity, 41, 56
LTK (laser thermal keratoplasy), 84
lupus, 25

M

magnifying glasses, 11
make-up, 56, 73
malpractice, 33
measurement
axis, 11
cylinder, 11
sphere, 10
Medi-Net, 34
medical
  associations, 27, 28
  history, 39, 40
medications, 53
menopause, 68
microkeratome
  corneal abrasion, 67
  history of, 15-17
  used in LASIK, 17, 52
mini-RK, 79
monovision, 48, 49
  correction, 83
myopia, 7, 10, 43
  see also nearsightedness
  correction with LASIK, 19
  increasing with age, 21
  outcomes, 61–63

N

National Board of Medical
  Examiners, 29
nearsightedness, 7, 10
  see also myopia
negative diopter, 11
nerve tissue, 6
  see also retina
night glare, 68, 69
  after photorefractive
  keratectomy (PRK), 77
night vision
  poor, 24, 48
nondominant eye, 48
nonfreeze keratomileusis, 15
nonogram, 30
nonsurgical vision correction
  options, 12, 13
normal vision, 6, 9, 10

O

Official ABMS Directory of
  Board Certified Specialists, 28
old eyes
  see prebyopia
ophthalmic boards, 27, 28
ophthalmologist, 26, 33, 47, 64
  qualifications for LASIK, 26–28
  referrals, 27
optic nerve, 6, 41
optometrist, 27
oral sedative
  prior to LASIK, 51
orthokeratology, 13
outcomes, 31–32

regression, 72
    after photorefractive
        keratectomy (PRK), 77
research activities, 74, 75
retina, 3, 6, 19, 41
retinal detachment, 83
retreatment with laser, 26
    see also enhancement
        procedure
returning to work, 44
(RGP) rigid gas permeable
    lenses, 39
rheumatoid arthritis, 25
rigid gas permeable (RGP)
    lenses, 39
risks, 44, 64–73
RK (radial keratotomy), 46
Ruiz, Dr. Luis, 15

S

"Sands of the Sahara" syndrome,
    72
scarring
    corneal, 13, 46, 85
sclera, 4, 85, 86
scleral expansion bands (SEBs),
    86
sculpting cornea, 18
screening, 64
SEBs (scleral expansion bands),
    86
sedatives, 54
side effects, 43
Snellen eye chart, 9, 20, 68
sphere measurement, 10
stable prescription, 22

star bursts, 24, 68, 69
statistics, 61–63
striae, 69, 71
    see also wrinkles
stroma, 4, 16, 17, 69
success rates
    with LASIK, 20, 32
suction ring, 51
sunglasses, 56
surgeon
    complication rates, 32
    consulting, 38–49
    credentials, 28–30
    finding, 26–28
    malpractice, 33
    number of procedures
        performed, 30
    procedures performed with
        same refractive error,
        30–31
    qualifications for LASIK,
        26–28
    questions to ask, 28–36
    referrals, 27
    reputation, 28
    research activities, 32
    success rates, 20, 32
    training, 36
surgically ideal eyes, 22
Swinger, Dr. Casimir, 15

T

tear duct drainage
    blocking, 45
tear supplements, 45
    see also artificial tears

About the Authors

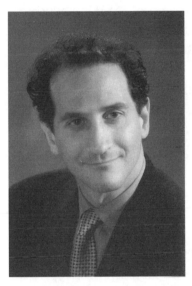

Ernest W. Kornmehl, M.D., F.A.C.S., is a board-certified ophthalmologist and medical director of the Kornmehl Laser Eye Associates in Boston. He completed his ophthalmology residency and chief residency at the Yale Eye Center, Yale School of Medicine, followed by a Heed fellowship in corneal surgery at the Massachusetts Eye and Ear Infirmary, Harvard Medical School. He also served as director of the Novatec Laser Surgery Program for Nearsightedness at the Massachusetts Eye and Ear Infirmary, Harvard Medical School. Dr. Kornmehl is a clinical instructor at Harvard Medical School, an associate clinical professor of ophthalmology at the Tufts School of Medicine, and a research associate at the Massachusetts Institute of Technology.

Dr. Kornmehl has taught surgery for nearsightedness and astigmatism at the American Academy of Ophthalmology (AAO) since 1987. He is a recipient of the AAO Honor Award for his numerous scientific presentations and instruction courses. He serves as an examiner for the American Board of Ophthalmology. Dr. Kornmehl also serves on the executive board and is a past president of the Massachusetts Society of Eye Physicians and Surgeons. He was also president of Boston Aid to the Blind and was appointed by the governor of Massachusetts to the Commission for the Blind.

Dr. Kornmehl is the developer of the Kornmehl LASIK System, specialized instruments used during the LASIK procedure. These instruments are used by refractive surgeons around the world and are manufactured by Akorn-Metico, one of the country's largest manufacturers of ophthalmic surgical instruments. Dr. Kornmehl is also co-developer of the S-K (Swinger-Kornmehl) solution, used to reduce corneal swelling.

Dr. Kornmehl lectures nationally and internationally, has authored numerous scientific publications and chapters in textbooks, and serves on the editorial boards of *Ophthalmology Times* and *EyeNet*, the official publication of the AAO. He has received several research grants from the National Institutes of Health and has recently developed a method of transforming skin into corneal tissue.

Dr. Kornmehl has been quoted in the *Journal of the American Medical Association, Health News/New England Journal of Medicine, Boston Globe, Family Circle, Good Housekeeping, Mademoiselle, Prevention* magazine, *More* magazine, and *USA Today*. He has been interviewed by WBZ-TV, WCVB-TV, WB56-TV, *CBS Evening News/Healthwatch, CNN, World News Tonight*, and the *Today Show*.

Dr. Kornmehl may be reached through his Web site: www.visionboston.com.

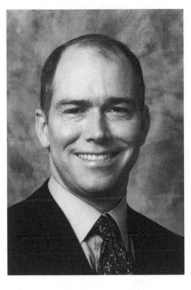

Robert K. Maloney, M.D., M.A. (Oxon), is the founder and current director of the Maloney Vision Institute in Los Angeles. The first surgeon to perform LASIK in western North America, Dr. Maloney was voted one of America's top ten vision correction specialists in a nationwide survey of eye surgeons.

A Rhodes Scholar, Dr. Maloney trained at Oxford University, Harvard University, and Johns Hopkins Hospital. While a professor at UCLA, he trained more than 700 surgeons in the use of the excimer laser. He has performed more than 20,000 LASIK surgeries and had LASIK performed on his own eyes in 1997.

Dr. Maloney has been invited to more than 100 lectures on five continents and has published more than 150 articles and abstracts. He received the Lans Award of the International Society of Refractive Surgery for his innovative contributions to the field.

Dr. Maloney's numerous broadcast appearances include NBC's *Extra*, ABC's *20/20* and *Prime Time Live*, PBS's *Life and Times*, and CNN's *The World Today*. He has been featured in the *New York Times*, *USA Today*, and the *Wall Street Journal*. He is also listed in *Who's Who in the World*, *Los Angeles Magazine's* "Best Doctors in LA," and Braun's *Best Doctors in America*. He is widely recognized as one of the leading refractive surgeons in the world.

Dr. Maloney may be reached through his Web site: www.maloneyvision.com.

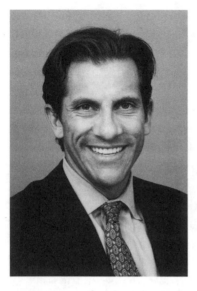

Jonathan M. Davidorf, M.D., is a board-certified ophthalmologist and Director of the Davidorf Eye Group in West Hills, California, where he specializes in laser vision correction and lens implant surgery. He is a member of the teaching faculty at U.C.L.A.'s Jules Stein Eye Institute, Director of Surgeon Training for Refractec, Inc., Chief Ophthalmologist for the Women's World Cup, and Co-Director of Friends of Vision Foundation, a nonprofit organization that provides medical and surgical ophthalmologic care to underdeveloped nations. Dr. Davidorf was an Academic All-American at the University of California, Berkeley; he continued his training at the University of California, San Diego, U.C.L.A., and Ohio State University. He completed an international fellowship in refractive surgery in South America, where he researched and helped develop LASIK and other refractive surgery techniques, several years before their approval in the United States.

Among his publications are the definitive scientific papers on implantable contact lenses and Bioptics vision correction surgery and pioneering work on pediatric LASIK. Dr. Davidorf is also co-author of *LASIK: Principles and Techniques*, the first medical textbook on LASIK. He has served as investigator for many clinical trials, including the investigations that led to FDA approval of LASIK. In 1999, Dr. Davidorf received recognition from the International Society of Refractive Surgery for best research by a vision scientist.

Dr. Davidorf has delivered award-winning presentations to national and international audiences on the subject of refractive surgery and continues to train other ophthalmologists on advanced surgical techniques. His course, "Emerging Technologies in Cataract and Refractive Surgery," is attended by surgeons from around the world. He is a lecturer and course director for the American Academy of Ophthalmology, the American Society of Cataract and Refractive Surgery, and the International Society of Refractive Surgery. His media appearances include news telecasts for ABC, CBS, NBC, and Fox. He has also been interviewed for numerous radio programs and has been featured in newspaper and magazine articles coast to coast.

Dr. Davidorf may be reached through his Web site: www.davidorf.com.